This new edition of Juliette's memoir has been edited for accuracy and clarity; new illustrations and photos have been added, making it substantially different from the earlier work of the same name published by Faber and Faber, London, England in 1955.

This jewel-like memoir by noted herbalist and traveler **Juliette de Bairacli Levy** details her personal struggle against typhus fever, during which she gave birth to her second child, Luz, who had to be suckled by a nanny goat. As ever, we are embraced by Juliette's love of nature and animals, and welcome onlookers as she relates with people whose lives are far different from ours.

Gypsies dance and sing their way through this book, adding their picturesque – and sometime threatening – energy to an exquisitely detailed story that is always intriguing, and sometimes suspenseful.

Juliette shares with us the herbal lore she learned and used in the Spanish Sierra Nevada mountains. You'll find herbs to combat vermin, counter burns, keep your skin beautiful, and many more.

Smell the cool waters of the mill stream; listen to the sounds of the goats and sheep as they climb the dusty roads; enjoy the flowers and the processions that make Spanish mountain life so colorful; and marvel at the ancient herbal wisdom that saves Juliette and her children, Rafik and Luz.

Praise for *Spanish Mountain Life*

"Juliette's gentle guidance helped me and thousands of others to awaken their souls to Nature."
Rosemary Gladstar, *Family Herbal*

"Juliette's voice is lyrical, even as she narrowly escapes death. Her indomitable spirit shines through."
Susun S Weed, *Healing Wise*

For
Rafik and Luz
who shared the
Spanish Mountain Life

Spanish Mountain Life

Juliette de Bairacli Levy

By **Juliette de Bairacli Levy**
from
Ash Tree Publishing
www.ashtreepublishing.com

Common Herbs for Natural Health
A Gypsy in New York
Nature's Children
Spanish Mountain Life
Summer in Galilee
Traveler's Joy

Spanish
Mountain
Life

Juliette de Bairacli Levy

with photos from the author's archives

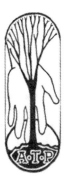

Ash Tree Publishing
Woodstock, NY

Ash Tree Publishing
PO Box 64
Woodstock, NY 12498
845-246-8081

www.wisewomanbookshop.com (to buy our books)
www.ashtreepublishing.com (to learn more about our
     books and authors)
www.susunweed.com (for more information on herbs)

Publisher's Cataloging in Publication
(Prepared by Quality Books Inc.)

Bairacli-Levy, Juliette de.
    Spanish Mountain Life / Juliette de Bairacli Levy.
    Rev. and updated ed.
    p. cm.
    Includes index.
    LCCN 2005934396
    ISBN-13: 978-1-888123-07-4
    ISBN-10: 1-888123-07-9

    1. Bairacli-Levy, Juliette de. 2. Herbalists–Biography.
    3. Materia medica, Vegetable. 4. Medicinal plants.
    5. Romanies–Spain–Social life and customs.
    6. Mountains–Spain–Description and travel.
    I. Bairacli-Levy II. Title.

RS164.B292 2006   615'.321'092
                         QBI06-600259

Table of Contents

List of Illustrations

I was without my camera during all my time on the Sierra Nevada. But friends have illustrated my book for me: Spanish, American, and Swedish. My grateful thanks to all. Also my thanks to my Welsh friend, Powell Jones, M.I.B.P., for his printing and enlarging. The Fiesta photo of Luz was taken after I had left the mountain.

J. de B-L.

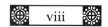

Herbal Index

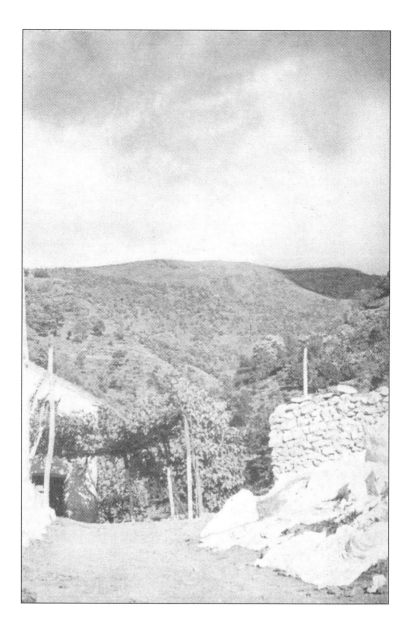

Sierra foothills beyond the water-mill.
Photo by Juan Mingorance

Chapter One

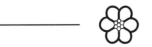

The Arrival

So vast a mountain is the Sierra Nevada range that it is a country in itself, with its towns and many villages, its rivers and streams, and the strange ways of the people who farm or trade or merely live there, and who truly preserve much of the ancient life of Spain.

This book tells only about the mountain life in the area of the water-mill where I lived from early spring to late autumn: Where my second child was born and I and my first child nearly knew entombment in the cemetery of Lanjaron as victims of the typhus fever which plagues that part of the Sierra Nevada.

I arrived in the small sierra town of Lanjaron in March. The town is a two hour bus ride from Granada. It has deserved fame for its medicinal springs in the far part of the town away from the Sierra Nevada towards the sierra of Montril. It is famous also for its orchards, cheeses, and the basket-weaving of the many Gypsies, who live in their own ancient quarters – *barrios* – of Lanjaron.

I stayed at first in an inn in the town center, overlooking the part of the Nevada range where it meets that of Montril. It was several weeks before I found my room and terrace garden in the old water-mill of Gongoras, at the foot of the Sierra Nevada, some miles from the town.

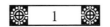

Spanish Mountain Life

That March the weather was bitter: the worst early spring that had come to Andalusia in fifty years. Much snow had fallen in Lanjaron, a rare thing in that town. The orange and lemon crops were largely spoiled, and all the upper ranges of the mountains wore cold white shrouds of deep frozen snow. Ravens screamed in the blue-white air, hungry for the blood of the newborn young of the sheep and goats which teemed on the mountain. The men wore thick woolen cloaks and broad-brimmed felt hats or tight berets, and the children's legs pricked uncomfortably in the unaccustomed wear of coarse, woolen stockings.

The cold kept the people indoors, and over the entire town hung a gauzy perfumed veil of rosemary smoke, that shrub being the chief fuel of Lanjaron and the surrounding sierra farms. Daily the men and boys – and sometimes the young women – collected great bundles of rosemary from the mountain-sides, and brought this fragrant fuel back to town on their horses, mules and donkeys, leaving a further scented trail as the rosemary brushed against the walls of the houses in the narrow ways.

Nearly every family in the town owned a transport animal, and many owned also goats, chickens, pigeons, and a pig or two. These animals were stabled, strangely, in the ground-floor rooms or basements of the houses. When I lived in the inn I was amused by a herd of goats which was stabled in a house facing my window. Every morning around seven o'clock the door was opened wide, and out into the street hurried forth an immense family of goats, fifty strong or more, of all sizes and colors, including many of the lovely blue-gray shade of wild lavender, a type of fine-horned goat much seen on the Sierra Nevada where, also, many wild goats live. For a reason beyond explaining, I was always reminded of the Pied Piper of Hamelin: and yet this was a going forth into the light, not an entry into the darkness of a mountain. Perhaps that thought came to me because of the music of the goat bells, which altogether seemed to produce a wild piping; and perhaps also I was influenced by the tall hat and the cloak of the youth who shepherded the flock.

"The goats! The goats!" always shouted my two-year-old son Rafik, in his shrill Spanish. He was daily at the window to watch them and the many other animals which made up the long morning procession to the mountain, where the snows melting beneath a cold wintry sun had given way in many places to stretches of sweet new grass, and there was leafage again on the bushes, and wild flowers among the rocks: hyacinths and cyclamens.

All alongside the many streams of the mountain there was also a flowering of many tiny things, such as scented violets, chickweed, red and yellow pimpernel, white clover, and in the water itself, much watercress which Rafik and I gathered for our midday meals. The winding roads of the mountain, later to become ankle-deep in white dust, were bordered by fleshy-leaved, gray-hued aloes and cacti.

The passing of the goat flock in front of my window was repeated by others throughout Lanjaron: Every morning house doors were opened to pass out animals of all sorts, hungry for the feed of the mountain. They were attended by men and youths, frequently Gypsies, either on foot or mounted on their donkeys, mules or horses, the latter very often colorfully decorated with harness and saddle trappings, the saddles being embroidered with bright wools and hung with fringes – which are also a deterrent to flies – of crimson and saffron wools, almost always only those two colors.

The music of that Sierra Nevada procession of animals! Collar and harness bells pealed, hooves beat wild on the modern concreted road, the herd dogs barked, and men shouted instructions to their mounts: "burr-o!" for their donkeys, "gall-arr" for their mules, and "hack-ah" the horses. The herding cry for the goats was always "she-bah, she-bah!" Otherwise the men were very silent.

But away by the streams of the three mills and the narrow river Husagre, the women sang as they washed their household linen and clothes; they gossiped much, also, one about the other. Washing on the mountains was very easy. Machines and soap powders were not needed. Exposure to the fierce sun bleached out all stains, and likewise dried out all moisture in quick time. Housework, too, was very easy. A sweep-out with an old-fashioned broom, then a wipe-over of furniture, with paper to remove dust, then a cloth moistened first with vinegar to erase marks, then polished with a little olive oil, made fragrant by having steeped in it, again in the hot sun, mountain flowers: lavender, thyme, or the strongly-scented blossoms of the broom.

The singing heard on the Sierra Nevada is typical Andaluz. The sweet and sad throbbing chant of flamenco, which resembles Moorish song, was doubtless influenced by the long occupation by the Moors of the Andalusian area of Spain facing Morocco.

The women and girls also go forth from the houses to the sierra; they to the nearer places to cut fodder for the immediate needs of the animals which have not gone out to graze, and to gather also herbs for their cooking, especially fennel and sorrel, sweet mint, a sweet watercress, water-celery and a form of wild onion of much abundance. Watercress is not very popular with them, and they scorn chickweed and nettles, all of which Rafik and I ate in a daily salad, especially the water-celery.

That going to and from the mountain of the people and animals was the heart of the life of that part of the Sierra Nevada. Every evening I took my child to meet the procession of the animals as they came home, for he loved the beasts of all kinds as much as I loved them, and that was very much indeed.

My greatest affinity was with the herbivorous creatures, especially the sheep, goats, cows, horses, camels, and the wild deer. On the sierra roads I met with an abundance of all – except the camel and deer, although the latter does live in some remoter parts of the mountain.

How good it was to be close to so many animals and all of them in fine health, excepting perhaps some of the cows, who suffered from mastitis, due mostly, I believe, to irregular milking and being walked long distances when their udders were unnaturally heavy with milk. Rafik and I liked to see the great herds, and have the sweet herbage scent of them, and touch their strong bodies with our hands. The goats especially came to know us, and would greet us in their high vibrant voices and nuzzle against us.

We also took walks on the mountain every morning, despite the cold of the Andalusian spring. The breath of the sierra wind was icy; snow and hail came in it often enough. It was colder than anything that I had known elsewhere in Europe, including the French Alps in February, or even during mid-winter on the sea-coast beyond Istanbul in Turkey. The Sierra Nevada peasants said: "This wind enters the heart of the bones," and they would wrap their woolen cloaks tighter around their lean bodies. But Rafik and I had no woolen clothes, for I had expected to find the hot Andalusian sun which I had known in the spring in Granada two years ago. We shivered in our thin clothes and were thankful when the evening brazier of olive-wood charcoal was lit in our room in the inn and we could warm away the cold of the day.

I could not forgo our walks despite the snow and rain, for all the terraced slopes of the fertile lower areas of the sierra were in blossom. Fruit trees of every kind seemed as multitudinous as the sierra animals, and the blossom lay lovely upon them, of all colors of white and pink, from the ivory of pear flowers to the darker rose hue of quince and almond, to the green-white, most fragrant blossoms of the orange and lemon trees. Trees in blossom, seen against a turquoise sky when the rains clear, are a fair thing. And, later, the carmine of pomegranate flowers against the blue was the loveliest of all.

I knew some sadness when all the snow melted on the sierra heights around Lanjaron; the eternal snow of the Sierra Nevada is on higher ranges, out of walking or mule-riding distance of the *molino* (mill) Gongoras. But with the melting of the snow came the wild purple irises, tall as Rafik, beautiful banners of them along the borders of the streams and waving upon the wet parts of the foothills. Their scent was a delight and I gathered armfuls of them for my room in the water-mill. They flowered at Eastertime, the Semana Santa of Spain, and the peasants told me that they represent the pain of Christ; certainly the purple iris was much used in the church processions of that holy week.

Later, the peasants also said that the white Madonna lily – the *azucena*, so celebrated in songs and dances of Spain – represents the happiness of Christ, His triumph over death, and that the white lilies would blossom when the irises had died away. And that was so. So soon as the irises had withered on the mountain, the madonna lilies flowered thick along the border of the upper mill stream of the molino Gongoras, and like the white of swans were reflected in the sunlit waters of the stream. They, too, had their turn in the church processions, especially the June celebration of *Corpus Christi.*

There blossomed also by the mill streams, white may, and on the near gray rocks a sweet variety of wild lavender. With these flowers came the nightingales. Not a mere one or two birds as in most parts of Europe, but a multitude, so that one seemed to sing in every bush. Oh the wild piping of them! by day and by night, though on the Sierra Nevada they sang – mostly by day, for the nights stayed cold that May month. Concerning the nightingales the peasants again spoke beautifully: "The *ruiseñores* have pearls and corals in their throats."

The sun of the day became very hot by May, and the flies bred rapidly. Those swarming flies! The curse of Lanjaron; carriers of disease, including the dread typhus fever. The flies are few around Granada, but all upon Lanjaron they swarmed, even reaching up into the high sierra above the town and far around to plague the people there on the remote farms. Many persons who came to drink the waters of the medicinal springs went away because of the flies. If the typhus fever had not kept me in Lanjaron I believe that I, too, would have fled from that insect plague.

The abundance of those flies is difficult to describe: I have only met with a near likeness around the town of Houmpt Souk on the island of Djerba, where they bred in thousands upon the open cesspits. In Lanjaron there were also most unsanitary conditions away from the clean part of the town – where the hotels for the visitors to the mineral springs were. That part was very clean and cool and well-kept. For the rest, the children piled their excreta in the back streets; and then the sierra animals which came nightly into the town further fed the flies.

I well recall two unpleasant things of the mountain town. The square opposite the inn where I first lived, brought to me the unsanitary and miserable life of the very poor, such as children shut out in the streets by drunken parents, and women picking from one another's heads teeming lice and their nits. The other unpleasant thing was a huge sow kept in the basement – so that the entire house smelt of the pig – in conditions of indescribable dirt. The animal itself was memorable for the black coat that it wore over-all; it was a cloak of flies! Except for snout and tail there was scarcely a centimeter of its gray-white body to be seen.

In the main street of the town the flies lay on roadway and pavement like black treacle, and likewise they gathered upon the walls of the houses and shops. The wares in the shops were invariably speckled black with fly excreta. Whether fruit or crockery, lengths of dress material or bread, all habitually bore the dirty imprints of the flies. It is difficult to wash fruit clean of such contamination without spoiling it and losing most of the flavor. Therefore, whenever possible, I bought my fruit direct from the sierra farms, or asked the shop-keepers to sell me fruit from the lower areas of the boxes and baskets, where the flies had not had entry. The flies made it impossible to open one's doors or windows by day; only late into the night until soon after dawn dare one do so.

To defy this rule of Lanjaron was to ensure the entry of a black hissing fly swarm into one's house, soiling everything, falling into water-jugs and milk, and at night-time descending upon the beds to crawl over the faces of the sleepers. They had the same fly habits as those of Arab lands; they liked to be upon the human body. Favorite places were the corners of the eyes and mouths of children from which they sucked moisture and at the same time left bacteria of disease. It was very general in Lanjaron to see babies' faces speckled with fly excreta.

The people nearly all possessed fly-swishes, which the Gypsies made and sold: a stout cane onto the top of which was wired a head of colored paper streamers. With this weapon one swished the flies out of one's home and back into the streets, and also away from one's body. But the fly swishing was not so easy so far as the house rooms were concerned. Through an opened door one tried to beat out the black hordes. But a large percentage of them went into hiding! As soon as the door was closed, out of their hiding places, beneath beds and in wall niches, they came, and danced in triumph before one's angry eyes!

What happened with those flies in my water-mill home during the three weeks when I had typhus fever and was half-insane and entirely unable to defend my room and my children against the hordes, I shall never know. Vast swarms of flies habitually hung around the mill. The fruit trees were blamed, the water was blamed, as was the flour in the mill. But, in truth, the dirtiness of the place was responsible. The mill family never seemed to notice the flies at all. They would sit placidly eating their meals, their faces, hands and clothes black-plastered with flies; also equally plastered was the food that they ate!

There had been few flies about on the mountain and in its town during the first months of the cold spring. They came with the sun just before I developed typhus fever. Then later the burning sun of the summer slew them, and by mid-September they were few. It was sad that they had been over Lanjaron during the time of the nightingales, so that I had never been able to sit in peace by day and enjoy the wonderful singing by the mill streams. But there were compensations! The beauty of the flowers was one. I especially loved a big and very old rose-bush by the upper stream. That red rose was named *terciopela* after Spanish velvet, and its red was so rich the hearts of the flowers were almost black of hue. The scent was magnificent.

I had a bathing place in the stream alongside the rose bush. There I could lie in the cold sweet water from the sierra, enjoy the scent of the roses, and at the same time hear the nightingales. This pleasure helped to keep me from death during the worst times of the typhus fever when my body was half dead and only my heart seemed to keep feebly alive.

Another compensation was the wheat. It was but a small green child at the time of my coming to the Sierra Nevada, and I watched it grow into golden adulthood. A field of wheat came right against my wall, and later, during my illness, the sheaves of the cut wheat — for it was harvested early over the sierra to make place for the following crop of maize — were piled on my white sun-drenched wall to dry and harden. How rich was the mountain of wheat! In green waves, and then in golden ones, it flowed over the countless terraces of the sierra: that old Moorish type of agriculture conserved the water of the rains, and the streams were diverted on the heights of the mountains to irrigate the lands of the farmers turn by turn. The wheat rustled like the crisp frilled gowns of the Gypsy dancers of Granada. Later I was to buy a sack of the almost copper-hued grain and had it ground into flour by the great mill-stone of the molino Gongoras; then I made it into bread for Rafik and me, and into a gruel for the baby.

Throughout my time at the water-mill the mountain was always my friend, giving always pleasing gifts for my eyes: changing hues as the seasons passed by, animals – lizards and serpents, myriads of butterflies and dragon-flies – and birds. At night its stars silvered everything with their brilliant light, and glow-worms lit their tiny lights in the mill garden by the upper stream and on the rocks of my terrace, even shining on the rocky wall of my room.

And then there was its music. The rustle of the fruit trees, grape-vines and crops, wheat and then maize, and the singing of birds and insects. Other than the nightingales there was a lovely piping bird which the peasants called "cuckoo"; but it was not a cuckoo at all, for it piped by night only and was not migratory, and stayed through the spring and summer, and did not steal the nests of other birds for its young. This "cuckoo" remained unseen; I never once saw it. To me it was the mysterious plaintive piper of the mountain. There were doves and pigeons on the high crests of the sierra, where the snow is eternal; there is a snow-plumed bird belonging to the Sierra Nevada, the rare paloma torcaza.

Then, at the time of the figs and grapes, there came another piper, this time by day, with such sweet music: the *colorina*, which in Tunisia is called the lark of Africa, and which I shall always associate with the shimmering date palms of the island of Djerba, where the *colorina* wove their love-flights over the huge fronds. Frogs also piped in harsh ugly voices, and kept tune with the singing insects: the *chicharra* insect which loved the wheat fields and the olive groves and made metallic endless zither music with its wiry wings; the huge crickets – *grillos* – and the tiny house crickets which sang in the chimney and cane rafters of my room.

In my room also were salamanders who croaked strangely and huge moths beating against the lamp. That was the sierra music by day and night. The miller's eldest son, Fraquito, told me a verse concerning the springtime music of the creatures of the Sierra Nevada, childish but true.

> *All the day the* chicharra *sings in the sun,*
> *In the midnight hour calls the* cuco,
> *At two in the morning the* tutuvia *whistles,*
> *At three chants the* ruiseñor,
> *At four twitters the* golondrina,
> *And at five comes the dawn!*

How true it was of the *golondrinas* – the swallows. I shall evermore associate them with those weeks when I was caring for Rafik when he, too, was ill with typhus fever. The young of the swallows used to gather on the wires of the tall grapevines to welcome the first dawn rays of the sun, and their twittering came loud into the room.

Their chorus calendared the advent of a new day of life for Rafik, and for myself: a new battle with death to keep my child from those insatiable hands which earlier had reached out passionately to take me also. The swallows gave me courage, and later the mountain gave us back our health.

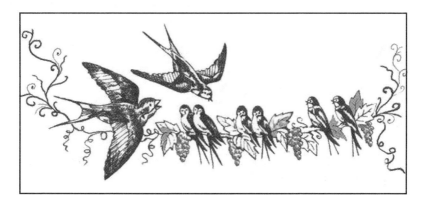

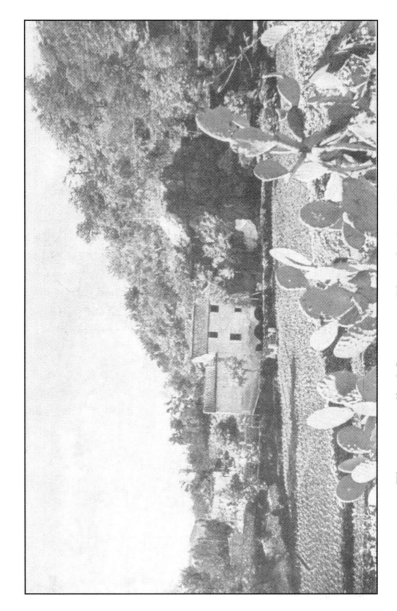

The water-mill of Gongoras. Photo by Juan Mingorance

Chapter Two

The Water-Mill

The water-mill of Gongoras is very old. When I asked the miller's sons what age was the mill, they spoke together only one word—*siempre*—always, forever. Since the beginning of agricultural life on the Sierra Nevada, the water-mill of Gongoras had stood strong and square, its wide feet quarried out of the sierra rocks, the rafters of its roof built of the surrounding trees, the chestnut and the olive. There is a famed Spanish poet named Luis de Gongora, but no one seemed to know if that had association with the mill, which was far older than the poet.

In the narrow verdant valley of the river Husagre there are three water-mills, standing one above the other, up the lower slopes of the sierra. Mountain waters roar around all three of them, and in the heat of an Andalusian summer noon, the mill pools are dark and cool. Only in the later months of summer, and reaching into the autumn, the waters of the molino Gongoras were fouled by women washing the intestines of animals for stuffing later with pig blood and meat. How strange are human beings! In the lovely months of August and September, so rich in fruits, cereal crops, and honey, they occupied their time with washing out intestines and gave no thought to their polluting of clean streams.

The molino Gongoras is tall and square, its gray stone structure painted with white lime. Its windows are few, and small for the size of the mill. The basement seems to grow up from the weather-thrashed gray rocks. In front of the mill is a cobbled court, shaded above with grape-vines which send out green-yellow tendrils over the red beveled tiles of the roof. A steep path-way up the rocks and rock-hewn steps lead to an upper terrace, built above the stable of the goat and donkey, and walled around with wooden boxes holding plants. Fine carnations of many colors and rich scent, double larkspur – the blue of the Andalusian sky – and bright geraniums. By the summer, all are scorched away, and only a few leafy stalks remain, until September, when a fair rose-hued lily, called the lamp of Saint Mary, blossoms. Beneath the boxes are many pots of further plants; some growing in chipped enamel chamber-pots – which I think was very illustrative of the miller's wife: flowers in chamber-pots!

The terrace leads into a small square-shaped room, which has a ceiling support of tree rafters, the round bodies of the tree being used entire; and beneath this, a canopy of maize canes held together by cords of plaited grass. There is a back door to this room leading into the main mill-house.

From the terrace there goes up a further steep path, and steps, to a garden, through which courses the upper mill-stream. On the near side of the stream is a vegetable garden bordered with flowers; on the far side rise great rocks, leading to craggy heights on which grow prickly pear cactus; and far up, a fair and singing grove of slender birch trees. On the highest rock, the Falanges had erected a cross of white wood. Wild doves would perch there and make their sweet music. When I came to live in the water-mill – in the small room which led from the terrace – I often sun-bathed on those heights and dined well off the chumbas, cactus fruits, of which I had grown very fond when in Mexico. For further fruits there was a small orchard, with peach and apricot trees, and above all, a border of quince trees along the mill-stream, which afforded the necessary shade for the garden when the burning days of late spring and summer came.

That stream is the life-blood of the water-mill. Down from it, at its ending, are three big tunnel-like pits through which the water rushes when the wooden trap-doors are raised. This water turns the big wooden wheels beneath the mill, and they in turn send up a great force of the water which works the three big grinding-stones. When the mill is grinding corn, the water beaten by the big wheels spurts up and out in cold fans of shining spray, and the mill is filled with the music of the splashing waters and the grinding stones. I could hear it in my terrace room.

During late August and September, I had the good music of the grinding-stones by night and day, as they transformed the wheat of the golden summer into flour, and, later, ground the maize. As the stones turned, the mill seemed to quicken and sing its ancient song of work, and was a far happier place when its long enforced idleness was ended. For little work came to the water-mills except following harvest-time. The many bakeries of Lanjaron mostly preferred to buy cheap bleached flour from merchants in the big towns, the people themselves sharing the modern taste for refined products. Only the Gypsies sought out the natural flour, and the peasants on the distant farms, who still baked their own bread.

However, the family Lopez of the water-mill Gongoras made good use of the flours which they ground. An almost daily dish for their midday meal was *migas*, a porridge made from either wheat or maize, or, sometimes, a mixture of both. This was prepared in a huge frying-pan over the brushwood fire of rosemary or chestnut branches and wood-wrack from the streams. The porridge was simply a coarse flour mixed with water, garlic-flavored olive oil, and much salt, cooked slowly over the fire. It was eaten very hot, with big raw onions and lettuces as large and round as cabbages, both from the mill-garden.

Rafik and I liked to enter the big grinding-room of the mill when the mill-stones were working. The scent of the newly ground flour was so good, and the place itself so cool – that old, long chamber of stone, with its surrounding water was, indeed, cold. Swallows nested in the rafters, and dropped their lime into the flour as it ground: perhaps that is why it had such a good taste!

The miller's two sons, Fraquito and Rafael, brought Rafik many a baby swallow to hold in his loving hands. He kissed their dark blue heads, and then they were sent back into their nests again. The miller's sons also wrote for me Spanish words, when I questioned them as to the spelling of this or that: They wrote with a stick upon the flour in the troughs, as one writes also upon the sand.

The present-day bread of Lanjaron was modern, but, even in the bakeries, it was prepared the old way: pounded in wooden troughs and then baked in the huge oven over ash of rosemary shrub. I think that it was the many bakeries which were mainly responsible for the lovely scent of rosemary which hung over the town. People from a nearby town of Orgiva told me that in the old days before the popularity of the mineral springs of Lanjaron and the cleaning-up of the town to make it fit for tourist trade, the place smelt so bad that the people of Orgiva used to prepare handkerchiefs with cologne to hold to their noses as they rode through Lanjaron on journeys to Granada.

Certainly some of the back streets stank; but I recall mostly the scent of rosemary in association with Lanjaron.

In the bakeries women could prepare bread for their own homes and then give it to the baker to bake for them, for a small payment. Big white potatoes, with much crude salt rubbed into them, and the delicious fat yellow sweet potatoes, *batatas*, which taste and smell like chestnuts, were also roasted there for the people. Few of the houses possessed ovens. Most had only a small charcoal-fed fireplace for cooking or, in the more primitive homes, an open fire of brush-wood.

The baking of bread was ancient custom, and so was the threshing of the grain which was later to feed the big grindstones of the water-mills. All around the town were ancient stone threshing-grounds of circular shape, and on the higher farms, smaller individual ones. Upon those stone places the ripe wheat or maize was strewn, and the grain then threshed by small horse- or mule-driven carts possessing many pairs of toothed wheels: a dozen, fourteen and sometimes more wheels, arranged in pairs.

The monotony of that endless circling of the small area beneath a burning sun! But it was enjoyed by the children of the men threshing their individual crops of wheat, for the children were given rides in the small whirling carts. Later the chaff was sifted from the grain by tossing it with big wooden forks. Each fork that I saw – and held – was hand-modeled of fine, old, mellowed wood; they are part of the ancient poetry of threshing, and of the grain, which would later come in sackfuls, roped to the backs of the animals from the threshing-grounds, to be made into fine flour by the water-mill.

From that stone-ground whole grain, the miller's wife made bread which smelled as sweet as roasted hazel nuts, and which truly throbbed with strong health from the rich, unspoiled Sierra Nevada earth, and the power of the abundant sun.

But, as modern times and ways robbed the mill – and millers – of most of their former work, the family Lopez sought other trades. The miller's wife, in her front room by the vine-roofed earth court, sold wine and sodas to people who passed by the mill on their way to the shade of the river Husagre, in its upper heights, and the lovely river swimming-pool.

The miller's two sons gathered *mimbres* (willow) to sell to the many Gypsy families of basket-makers. Every May-time, when the willow was young and supple, a family of Gypsy basket-makers came to the mill and made baskets for the mill people. For food and wine, and some bundles of *mimbre,* they worked for nothing. In a day, three workers made four big baskets, and also two tiny miniature ones for the children: one for Rafik, and one for the daughter of the miller's elder son.

The baskets were fine pieces of work; the biggest one could hold a year-old child. They were lidded (to keep out the flies!) and most artistically woven in a trellis pattern. At this same time, the father of the family, and the most skilled worker, wove fine cane into the sides of Rafik's open carriage, a needed addition for my journeys to and from the town; also, I felt that a Gypsy-work carriage would mean good fortune for the baby when she was old enough to leave my arms and ride with Rafik.

There was a tradition at the mill that on the night of the festival of St. Juan, the 24th day of June, the Gypsies should come there to dance and sing. I had much looked forward to this, but it proved a night of bitter sadness. Firstly, very few Gypsies came, and not a guitar, mandolin, or other musical instrument among them. The present miller's wife – Patrocinio Gutierrez Gallardo Lopez – was not popular with the Gypsies and thus few came. I had entrusted the baby, Luz, to Patrocinio's care while first I, and then Rafik, battled typhus fever, and she had not known how to care for her.

The night of St. Juan, and the following night, was a crisis in my baby's life. The doctor told me that she would not live; but I willed that she would, that she would stay with Rafik and me. I used for her all the powers of herbal medicine, in which I have absolute faith. And the Gypsies prayed for her. She lived. I write more of the Gypsies in Chapter Six.

It was a strange thing that in my terrace room at the mill, I had a large colored print of St. Juan as a boy shepherd with a lamb in his arms. I had entered into occupation of the room to find the walls, hitherto bare, thronging with ghastly prints mostly of a religious nature, but so ill-printed and the characters depicted so ugly, that they were almost caricatures. I did not know how to rid my room of those pictures without insulting the feelings of Patrocinio. But one by one, using various quite flattering excuses, the pictures went away. I felt that I had to retain one, and there remained a colored print of an effeminate-looking priest holding a child, who in turn held white lilies.

Then, when Patrocinio escorted us through her rooms to see the swallows' nests above the grinding-room of the mill, I saw a picture I liked, and asked if I could change it for the priest and child! Patrocinio agreed promptly, and I thus gained quite a pleasant picture for my room. I always thought that the boy with halo and lamb was the child Jesus, and taught Rafik so. We came to like that picture very much, and often hung branches of flowers around its frame, the type of flowering branches that a shepherd boy would like to have. Not until Luz's recovery, following the night of St. Juan, did Patrocinio inform me that the picture was of St. Juan, who had once shepherded sheep.

It seemed the night of St. Juan always brought good fortune to the water-mill. Fraquito, too, had once been dying on that night: his trouble being gangrene of the knee from an infected leg wound. (The water-mill of Gongoras was certainly not a healthy place.) He, too, recovered following St. Juan's night.

Many a strolling player came to the water-mill during that summer. They knew that while I was at the mill there would always be glasses of wine forthcoming in reward for music or songs. Most of the players were Gypsies, but not all. The most memorable of them was a half-Gypsy singer from Casablanca. His mother was a Spanish Gypsy, his father French and without Gypsy blood. The singer was accompanied by a Spanish Gypsy guitarist, very accomplished, but ugly, like a vulture of face and skin, and his head bald of hair.

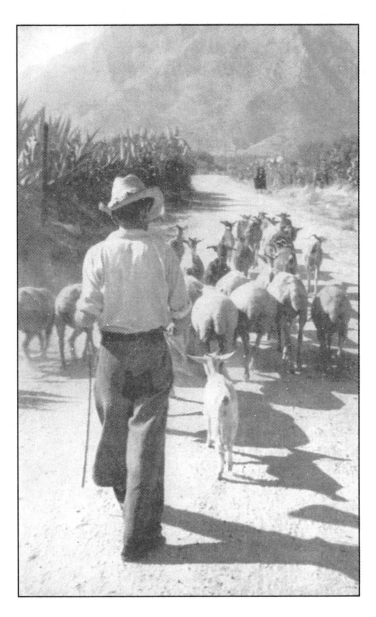

Typical flock on the hot dusty road to the mountain.
Photo by Paul Stephenson

He was the first, and only, bald-headed Gypsy that I have ever met during all of my travels and life with the Romanies. The singer was youthful, rather plain and over-small of face, but possessing a beautiful and finely molded nose typical of the Gypsies of southern Spain, his voice wonderfully powerful, and yet very sweet. He sang a Sevillano type of flamenco, his notes rising with the seeming power of a hundred skylarks.

The baby Luz kept her wide gray eyes upon the singer from Casablanca; she never stirred them, and her cheeks were very pink. She had been crying when the players had come to the water-mill, and I felt sure that I should not be able to enjoy the singing at all. But, as soon as I descended from the terrace and seated Luz facing the singer, she hushed her lament and her face glowed with pleasure. The young half-Gypsy singer was undoubtedly Luz's first love (at the age of four months!).

I told this to the singer and he laughed, pleased, and turned the flashy rings, with their bright artificial stones of glass, around on his fingers. He said that all of his songs would be for Luz, and he kept his pale blue eyes upon her gray ones as he sang; and the baby never moved throughout the singing and the very vibrant music of the guitar so close to her. I think she has a special love for the Gypsies. My long book about my travels with them had been much in my thoughts before her birth, being very recently published. Rafik, too, has been much with the Gypsies since his early months, and he loves them. What child would not love such people? None, unless they had previously been made afraid by adults' stories of Gypsy child-stealers and Gypsy witches! The Gypsies, with their bright clothes and jewelry, their dogs and horses, music and songs, frightened some and inspired others, especially the Spanish dancers. Gypsies come into the often drab world of a child like a flock of the bright birds of Paradise.

The days of summer passed away with sad swiftness. I, absolute lover of the sun, would have kept those summer days by me forever.

The terrace of the water-mill was made beautiful with the summer harvest drying there in the oven-hot sunlight of the late summer. Against the wall the neighbor now stacked sheaves of maize with their shining leaves and the auburn-tasseled fat cobs. The miller's wife spread out on the roof to dry over a hundredweight of tomatoes and black figs. The drying of the figs was a simple thing: they were merely picked fresh from the surrounding sierra trees and spread out upon layers of cane.

The tomatoes, too, were spread upon canes, but they had to be prepared. The head ends of the fruits were snicked open with a sharp knife, so that the fruit opened out like a crimson star-fish. Salt was then sprinkled over them to keep away the flies and wasps, and the tomatoes were left to dry for five days or so. I have never before eaten dried tomatoes – and how delicious they are. I dried fifty pounds of them myself for winter use.

Rafik was troublesome with those tomatoes. He loved to feast upon them, and would creep to where they were and stuff his mouth with them despite the salt which was spread thick as frost upon them. Then, all the day he thirsted for water. I had to invent stories to give him a distaste for that salty fruit, and in time he was very good, and those that he wished to eat he would bring to me to wash away the salt before the eating.

I saw snakes slithering across the terrace, and I feared for my baby, as her cradle was mostly upon the ground, either beneath the shade of the quince trees or in the long grass by a peach tree, which also gave shade and dropped its fruits into the cradle! I packed the cradle with garlic cloves beneath the mattress, and the heat of the sun brought out the pungent scent of that plant. I knew well that Gypsies use garlic to keep away vampires, and my aunt, Esther, of the old Egyptian family of Shushannah, had told me that the pearl-fishers of Aden strewed garlic in front of their shacks to keep away the great water-serpents. Her brother had been a pearl-trader and he had advised her about the garlic.

The Sierra Nevada has a strange belief concerning serpents. As I possessed a young baby, the belief was told to me many times, not only by peasants but by educated people who had been to school where such beliefs were usually scoffed away. I was told that mothers who have milk for young babies are likely to have their milk stolen from their breasts by serpents. The mountain snakes are very skilled in this theft of milk. They are said to insert their tails into the mouths of the babes. The babes suck the tails in contentment and the snakes feed from the mothers who believe that they are feeding their babes. This is always said to take place during the late night or early morning hours when the mothers are sleepy. When a group of people first told this legend to me at the river swimming-pool I scorned that any mother would be so stupid as not to distinguish the cold creeping body of a snake and its small hard mouth upon her body as compared to her baby.

But Isabel, who collected the bathing fees at the gate of the pool, assured me that her cousin's child had sucked a snake's tail for many nights before the snake was discovered. The child was very ill for weeks with swollen lips – which always occurred from having a snake's tail in his mouth – but later fully recovered. I usually spoiled the story by saying what was truthful: that I had no milk for my baby. Another thief had stolen that away: typhus fever. But the mother-scarers were not to be vanquished so easily. They invariably declared that nevertheless the baby smelt of the goat's milk on which she fed and the snakes, having a lust for milk, might well bite her.

Spanish Mountain Life

Perhaps I was impressed by that story, for I know from experience, in the mountains of Galilee, that snakes do like milk. Therefore, dismissing the first belief concerning the snake's tail, and accepting the second, I packed Luz's cradle with garlic heads from the mill garden, and tied there a necklace of blue wooden beads – the Turkish charm against the Evil Eye and habitually worn by children and animals in that land – which the Granada Gypsies had given to me as a gift for Rafik some time ago.

The springtime cherry harvest on the land of the watermill gave place to apricots and then peaches. There was a fine apricot tree alongside the cemetery wall, which was close by the water-mill. The fruits piled ungathered on the ground; people would not eat from that tree because of its nearness to the cemetery. One old sierra woman who came to the water-mill with a sack of maize for grinding told me that she had half her family in the near cemetery, and that after she had visited there she could never eat for two days, but only drank fennel water to drive away the unease from her body and soul.

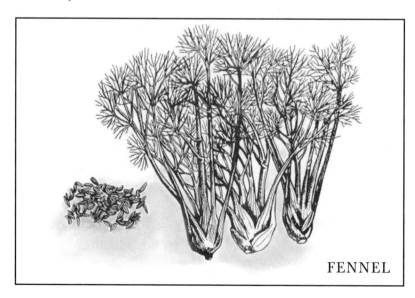

FENNEL

Then finally came the quince harvest, the richest of all. The trees which had flowered around the time of my coming to the water-mill were so heavy with the big hard fruits of delicious scent that their branches touched Rafik's corn-colored head as he raced to and fro beneath them. Great winds came with the quince harvest and blew dusty earth over everything. I had to go to the fountain to wash the fruit, for the stream of the water-mill was polluted by women washing intestines for their winter household sausage-making. Rafik bathed in the fountain, which belonged to the water-mill and was, I think, its most precious possession. I carried back a bucketful daily for the baby's bath; and I myself, during that time, went to a small waterfall in the upper river Husagre, where the water was unspoiled by humans.

We did sometimes paddle in the upper mill-stream when the days were especially hot, choosing the cleanest place, where the water came out through a dark grotto formed by the rocks. It was partly cleansed by the emergence from beneath the rocks, and was always very cold. The animals – birds and beasts – knew, too, that that was the cleanest place. The birds drank there, and a fat, stocky little animal resembling a water vole made its home in the mud, and would spoil the tranquility of our paddling by leaping from beneath our feet, always at unexpected moments.

The wind brought rain.The terrace outside my room became a pitch of mud: the roof leaked far worse than during the rains of early spring. As instinctively as the swallows, I have always known the time to go to a place and the time to leave. The autumn days commenced to shorten and the swallows gathered on the wires of the grape-vines and on ledges of the mill walls. I decided that I would leave with the swallows, although we were going to different places: they to the east, I to the north-west.

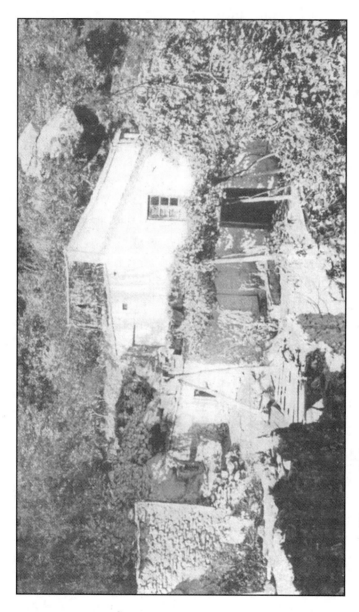

Water-mill showing terrace room with old flower boxes in foreground; above, the channel of the millstream. Photo by Juan Mingorance

Chapter Three

The Miller's Wife

Of the family Lopez of the molino Gongoras, the miller's wife was the chief actress; the others indeed were but small-part players. The miller's wife was everything: heroine, hero, and villain – very much villain.

My first meeting with Patrocinio Gutierrez Gallardo Lopez was memorable. It was during my early days in Lanjaron when I was living in the town inn. I was on my way to the swimming-pool, despite the bitter weather of that day, for I love to swim in icy water. I met with a stout, strong-bodied woman of medium height and middle age, clad in a rather fusty black gown. I was interested in the hardness and determination of the very pallid face; the flesh and the expression seemed to have much of the qualities of the gray rocks bordering the path, and which kept back the coursing, pushing waters of the river.

The woman told me that she knew of a short path to the swimming-place and which passed in front of her water-mill. So I went with her, along a rough, slippery path, then much flooded with water, which was a nuisance, as I had Rafik with me and soon his feet were very wet. We came to a part of the path which was impassable due to the floods of melted snow from the mountain in front of us. Patrocinio told me that we must cross the river and thus get back to the former road to the pool to which I had been walking when I met with her.

That was typical of her. She was always afterwards complicating my life in small things and big. She thereupon took Rafik up into her arms and skillfully leapt the slippery rocks, calling to me to follow, her voice peculiar and hoarse as a man's.

I could not follow. My leather sandals were slippery, and a fall on the rocks would surely mean a broken leg, or arm, and also, my second child was to be born in less than two months.

"Come on! Come on!" taunted the miller's wife.

A group of women were washing their linen nearby in a stream alongside the river. They told me not to attempt the river, concluding their advice with the warning concerning Patrocinio.

"She will do you no good! no good!" And that was what I was to hear from almost every person who spoke with me concerning Patrocinio, throughout my stay in Lanjaron.

But I considered the woman's leap across the river a feat to be admired. I took off my sandals and waded across to where she stood with Rafik in her broad arms. I accepted her invitation to visit the water-mill after I had had my bath in the pool.

I liked the old mill at once when the miller's wife showed me over it. I turned my eyes away from the family's dirty living quarters. What I liked was the age of the mill and its strength, the music of the waters which coursed around it, and the land and garden with its flowering fruit trees. The small terrace room was unoccupied. Rubbish was piled there, also, heaps of onions and old clothes. But I saw how it could be: cleaned and painted, with the boarded windows freed to let in more light and air.

In the room could be heard the music of the mill-stone then grinding, and also, faint as the whisper of sea in a coiled shell, the waters of the stream which sounded down the wide chimney from the other terrace above. Big fires of rosemary and olive-wood could be lit in the wide fireplace, and a person could sit in the sunlight in the doorway and please the eyes with the beauty of the sierra facing the terrace garden. I decided abruptly that it was the sort of primitive place which I would choose for the birth of my second child. My first had been born in an old Arab house on the lands of the Sheik of the island of Djerba, in Tunisia, who had given me his friendship. The dark hands of an old black midwife had been the first ones to hold Rafik. I told the miller's wife that I would like to live in her terrace-room. She agreed readily although rather surprised at my request. Thus I came to live in the water-mill and came also to know very well the remarkable Patrocinio.

In appearance the miller's wife much reminded me of another memorable personality whom I had come to know on my travels – the Algerian Gypsy sorceress, Primavera Heredia. The same ungainly body without waist, very wide hips and small head, which gave to her the appearance of a tortoise: the small head above the wide body, the head joined by a scraggy neck. The skin of the face was very loose and wrinkled, bloodless, gray-yellow; the eyes small and narrow and very deep-set, the iris of no marked color, brown-black and flaring red when angry; the teeth chipped, yellow, with fang-like canines, very strong for they could bite easily through the hard-wood of outer shells of almonds, for example; the hair center-parted, black with wiry strands of gray, all kept greased with olive oil; the voice very loud and male-like, her favorite cry being a loud "a-hoo, a-hoo," for surprise, pleasure and displeasure. Her step was swift in comparison to the ungainly body, and most silent, so that she was always surprising me with visits when I did not expect – and often did not want – to meet her.

But the badness of which her neighbors spoke, I truly did not find until, perhaps, the end of my days with her. The thing which annoyed and disappointed me most was that she considered all of my possessions to be her rightful own! What she took I will not state, but no matter how kind she was to me –

and she could be truly kind – the knowledge that she pilfered made me unable to like her very well. It became quite a game for me, though often a wearisome one, of hiding things where the miller's wife would not find them, though mostly with almost clairvoyant powers, she found all, and took again.

In shopping for me, she very often over-priced and under-weighed. But that I accepted, for she was such an excellent shopper. Just as a Gypsy knows the country-side, where the best things grow, so the miller's wife knew the town shops and the surrounding farms, and where to purchase the things which I needed. She was a natural forager, and foraged not only for her family, but for me also. Although she took my things – and I think it was beyond her self-control not to do so – I am sure she tried to atone for this by bouts of generosity and kindness. She was naturally generous, and perhaps she took in order to satisfy her pleasure in giving things and finding things. Whenever I lost anything she could almost always tell me where it was to be found.

Rafik and I lived mainly on white cheese of goat or ewe milk, home-baked wheaten and maize bread, goat milk and honey and an abundance of fruit. Every morning during mid- and late-summer Patrocinio brought to my room a plateful of figs and fruits of the prickly pear cactus, which she herself, despite her girth, had climbed trees and mounted the slippery weather-worn rocks of the sierra in order to gather.

She asked only pesetas the value of two shillings a week for that lovely fruit produce, and took nothing at all for tomatoes and peppers from the mill garden. It was at her suggestion that I purchased from a neighbor a big peach tree for a little less than one English pound.

What a joy that tree proved to me. The fruit was variety "Canary," globes of solid gold with crimson hearts. I think I would gladly have paid the pound just to have those golden globes crowding and tossing against the cornflower blue sky of Andalusia: for I took the fruits from the tree only as I needed them, and therefore for one month the gold tossed against the blue and I could watch this from the door of my room.

Patrocinio liked to collect fruit for me from my tree; it was the foraging instinct again, and I always gave a portion to her. But she took also! I found her hiding-place, a pile of my peaches beneath handfuls of grass where she was to come back for them later. I removed them all and replaced the grass. I had not the time to spare to stay within sight to see the expression on the face of the taker when she discovered her spoil had been taken likewise. It was petty of her, for she knew well she could have had, for the asking, as many peaches as she wanted. But I imagine that there was less excitement for her that way.

A quality of hers which I much admired was her knowledge of herbs, which she used much in cooking, in protecting the mill from evil visitants, and finally – and most importantly – as medicine. In Patrocinio I met a true fellow herbalist.

My first meeting with this medical knowledge of Patrocinio was when I developed a stiff neck due to the icy sierra winds of the early spring blowing through the open window-holes of the walls of the terrace-room. She took a thick piece of brown paper, made it very hot over the brush-wood fire, then applied on the paper a paste of rosemary charcoal and olive oil. This paper she placed around my throat, held in place by a strip of sheeting.

But this first medical treatment for me was not a success. The paper broke in the night, and during the early morning hours I awoke to find myself lying on a pricking heap of greasy powdered charcoal which blackened all of the bed linen around and also my body.

Her two most successful treatments were for a scalded arm and a prolonged fever. The arm was again treatment for myself, the fever cure was for Rafik during typhus. The scalding was memorable and terrible. It was during my own time of typhus fever which I developed in its most severe form.

I feel it a great defeat for an herbalist to be ill at all, but the transverse position of my baby in my body for seven months before her birth reduced my always strong health to a very weak state indeed. Plus, Rafik and I drank, for a month, polluted water from the upper mill-stream, due to the assurance of Patrocinio that the water was pure. This brought typhus to us, for typhus in Spain is not dependent upon lice as a carrier. People from the town washed their clothes, very possibly from typhus homes, in the nearby river and many times the river water came up into the mill streams.

The scalding was my entire right arm. Patrocinio had brought to my room a rubber water-bottle of boiling water to warm the baby's cradle before she was put to sleep there. The time was semi-dusk, and I was also half-stupid with the typical mental delirium of typhus. I did not see that the bottle was open, and pressed it to me to enjoy the heat. It poured out its contents over my arm. The May nights were cold and I was wearing a woolen jersey which held the boiling water against my flesh.

I remember hearing my voice screaming as if far from my body: "Patrocinio! Patrocinio! I've burnt my arm away. Come quickly! quickly!" The pain was overwhelming. Bad scalding is a great pain. The previous year I had kicked over a kettle of water which I had left on the floor. My foot had been badly burnt and I had been ill for several weeks.

Patrocinio applied at once her remedy to my scalded arm. She first well soaked the flesh in vinegar and then, a half-hour later, applied a thick paste of crude honey from the sierra which I always kept in my room, being a daily food for my children and me. The honey was renewed every hour and the arm kept covered beneath a piece of cotton cloth. Recovery was immediate. After only three honey applications all the pain had gone from my arm, which hitherto had felt as if a hundred fires were burning upon and within it. And although the scalding was wide – from near the shoulder joint to the wrist – in four days the cure was complete: There was not a mark to be seen on the arm, and I was able to end the honey treatments.

It was an interesting fact that I had wanted to apply my own herbal remedy of raw potato juice, which I had learned in Mexico, and used successfully, for example, on my foot. Patrocinio had lied to me that there were no potatoes obtainable, whereas later I noted that there was a field of them planted opposite the water-mill. She lied also that her son Rafael had been equally badly scalded on his leg and had recovered in a week and no scars left. But Rafael's true story concerning his scalding was that he had been left very ill and lame for many months and the scald area that he showed to me was permanently and badly scarred.

Patrocinio had lied for my own good: to prevent me from wanting treatment other than her own, in which she had justifiable faith. The potato juice of my own remedy had healed my foot, but very slowly. The honey cure was very rapid indeed.

I well recall the evening, during my early weeks in the water-mill, when a most peculiar and suffocating smell came seeping into my room. It was the work of the miller's wife! When I asked her the reason for this she told me she was driving out possible serpents, bats, and other beasts which may have lodged in the water-mill during the winter.

She had true reason to fear serpents in the mill, for later that summer I saw two at different times, fleeting across the mill terrace as I approached. And Rafik and I saw a very large one sunning itself close by the neighboring water-mill across the river. Patrocinio said that the niches in the nearby cemetery buildings were thronged with serpents.

She was using vegetables and human hair, she told me, and the burning was confined to the grinding-room of the mill. It seemed to me remarkable that, from so far away, the fumes should almost have suffocated me in my room. I felt that the stuff would be useful to advise in my veterinary work to fumigate byres, stables, and kennels where disease and vermin were present.

So I asked Patrocinio to tell me how she made the fumigation. She did: Twists of dried garlic stalks, enmeshed in human hair – animal hair would not work the fumes well – all sprinkled with dried *piquante* (small, very hot, red peppers), and a handful of powdered sulphur added to every three handfuls of the other matter, the whole then set alight.

But in the grinding-room, against the old rafters of the roof, were many nests of swallows with young already within.

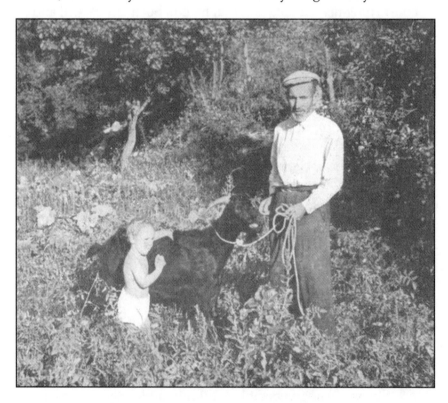

Rafik with the miller and Salud the goat.
Photo by Juan Mingorance

"What of the swallows?" I asked the miller's wife.

"They flew away when the fumes came."

"But their young ones! They will be suffocated for sure."

"The parents can make more."

Make more! She spoke that way again, later, when the baby Luz was very ill. There were many occasions when I had reason to dislike her: but all others I came to know on the Sierra Nevada were my friends.

I do not really know my feelings concerning Patrocinio. I would have been sad to have missed knowing in my life so strange and formidable a woman. And I did like many of her characteristic qualities: her ever-present sense of humor and her optimism. Flies were nothing, fleas were nothing and being near to death was nothing, all would dry up in the heat of the sun of Andalusia – flies, fleas and death!

I liked her for being a fellow herbalist and I loved her strange knowledge of portents and omens. She proved to be right always. Three examples: Before the birth of my child she told me to hold out one hand to her. I did so, my palm was upwards; she said the child would be a girl. If my hand had been turned palm downwards she would have known the child to be a boy. A girl was born.

A bluebottle fly one morning entered my room and disturbed everything with its abominable noise. Patrocinio told me that its entry at that hour meant that, within four days, I would receive a letter from my husband, Francisco Lancha Dominguez, a journalist who was away working on a Spanish-Arab journal in Tetuan. Francisco had not written me for a while, there was not at that time any particular reason why he should write, we both disliked composing letters in French which was the language which we both used, I speaking more French than Spanish. But on the fourth day exactly, there came a letter from Francisco.

One day, during the typhus fever, I had been lying in the sun, my wasted body drinking in its wonderful force, and as

I put on my dress again, a bee stung me between the shoulder blades. Patrocinio told me that I should be pleased for it was a sure sign that Francisco would be with me within two days. A visit from my husband was expected, but not so soon, and again no real reason why he should arrive at that particular time, but on the second day, Francisco was with me in Lanjaron.

She was well informed, too, concerning primitive rites of death. Much of what she knew was fearful. Two of the more pleasant things concerned the Moors and the Gypsies. Patrocinio recalled the burial of many Moors on the sierra during the Spanish civil war. They were not interred in the Catholic cemetery, but had graves away on the sierra, loaded with the traditional stones; the stones being there for two reasons, I believe: to keep out dogs and jackals (the latter in Arab lands), and to restrain the wandering spirits of the dead. The miller's wife said that every Moorish grave had interred with the body a bottle of wine, bread and fruit; doubtless again in consideration of the spirit.

"During those lean times of the civil war were not the graves sometimes plundered for the wine?" I asked.

"A-hoo! No! Everyone's too afraid of ghosts; anyway there's always wine to be had on the sierra come war or plague."

Of the Gypsies, she told of their fleeing a house whenever there came a death. It was house-dwelling Gypsies that she spoke of, as are most on the Sierra Nevada. Her information came out when I made my frantic declaration – with my baby nearly crossing the frontier away from our world – that if she died I would not remain in the water-mill one further hour, but would go away, far, immediately. And none would benefit from one possession of the baby, from earrings – by Spanish custom Luz had had her ears pierced when under one month old, and she wore tiny drop rings with brilliants and a blue Granada stone which matched the Andalusian sky and toned well with the child's sweet gray eyes – to cradle, I would burn it all.

"There you are again!" stated Patrocinio, "full of Gypsy ways. They do just as you've said now, the moving and the burning. They change houses even if it's only moving into each other's homes, perhaps next door, or even different rooms of the same house."

The miller's wife was a good wife and mother. She worked hard for her family, with the exception of keeping her house clean. The mill was filthy, for she disliked housework. I warred daily with her in order to have her clean my room properly. The door from my room which led into the mill I kept bolted, and all the many cracks sealed up with paper so that none of the uncleanliness should have entry. I told Patrocinio that the door was sealed against the flies which she allowed to swarm in her rooms.

I never heard her quarrel with the miller, and rarely with her children. But then the miller was a truly good man, if over-weak with his wife, letting her do so many things of which I know he did not approve. All spoke well of the miller and his eldest son, Fraquito, and I liked them both, except when Fraquito was bullying the goat. But I never knew them well, Patrocinio dominated so completely the stage of the watermill. Her only rival was the great wheel itself which made its powerful music as it turned and turned, and in its own way controlled the fortunes of the family.

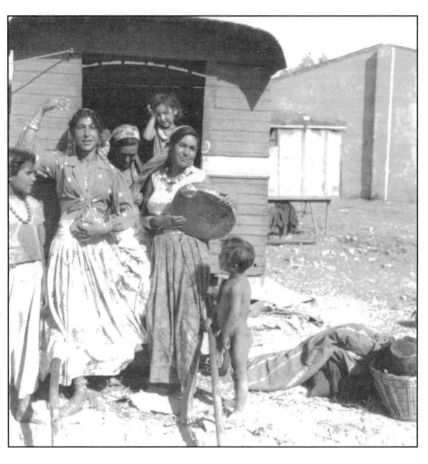

Spanish Gypsies at home in their caravan.
Photo by the author

Chapter Four

Typhus

Hitherto I had always associated typhus fever with squalor and overcrowding in places far from Europe, especially in China and India. Spain and typhus had never been together in my mind. How wrong I was! Typhus even has a part in Spanish history.

The old Spanish name for the fever was *tabardillo*, from the word for a red cloak, inspired by the crimson body rash which is one of the symptoms of epidemic typhus fever. Some of the old people of the Sierra Nevada still call the fever by that name.

The disease was brought to Spain as long ago as the fourteenth century, by soldiers returning from Cyprus. At the siege of Granada, later in the fifteenth century, typhus was an important factor in aiding Spanish victory, as the fever became epidemic among the Moorish defenders and slew more of them than any other weapon of war. So, I find that the immortal palace of the Alhambra of Granada has association with typhus fever. It is a strange fact that the severe form of typhus which was in Lanjaron when I was there, was said to have been brought over from Spanish Morocco by a Moorish family who had journeyed to Lanjaron to take the cure at the medicinal springs.

When I came to Lanjaron I took no precautions against that fever; I never thought of it at all. Perhaps I was over-confident concerning my health. I had long been convinced that if I lived truly close to nature I never would be ill. Again and again I had been given proof of this when exposed to infectious diseases during my travels. I knew that I was very rich in one possession which I valued most of all: powerful health.

But the critical transverse placement of my baby for the seven months before her birth depleted my health more than I had thought possible, and typhus came to me in its most severe form.

This fever is not always conveyed by vermin such as lice and bugs; one form can be carried by personal contact or typhus-polluted water. In this case it was the water of the mill-stream, polluted by the townspeople, which brought the fever. I repeat, I never thought of typhus; I knew only that a fever had developed and was making me very ill.

I fasted from all food, and expected that each day would end the fever: but it strengthened as I weakened. After one week of the fever there came another defeat: I had to cease feeding my milk to the baby and give her, instead, milk from the water-mill goat. I had hoped to feed her for a year, as with my first child; good health then had made that very easy.

The baby fretted at being deprived of her birthright: her mother's milk. Life abruptly became very bitter, whereas before the fever it had been joyous. My birthing had been accomplished most easily, without a doctor, only helped by the old Spanish midwife from the mountain. And it was a great happiness to me to possess a son and daughter, both of them affectionate and lovely to my eyes.

Around that time a mental stupor, which is one of the most horrible symptoms of typhus, came over me. The name "typhus" comes from the Greek word for mist or fog, refer-ring to the mental condition which is typical of that disease. I was robbed of three weeks of my life. The robber was, for me, a repulsive figure, with a bald head and cavernous face, a blood-red cloak hanging in folds around his skeleton-like body and reaching to his feet, which were swollen. How strange that, at an early stage of the typhus, I should have pictured a figure so true to the later stages of typhus fever. For the disease reduces the human body to a living skeleton very often, and later the hair, scorched like grass deprived of water on a sun-burning plain, dies and falls, leaving the head quite bald, both for women and men. Swollen hands and feet are, again, typical.

I cannot remember those three weeks of alternate stupor, delirium and near-normal mental state. During the normal times I cared for the children and even took them out for walks on the mountain-side, for neither I nor anyone else knew that I had typhus; at the water-mill they only saw that I was rather ill. It was only when I began to fall to the ground in weakness that the miller's wife, frightened, brought a doctor to the mill. The doctor, Americo Jiminez Moran, declared that I had a very advanced and severe fever. Coming so soon after the birth of my child, he did not think it possible for me to survive it. My husband and parents must be sent for.

At first I would not give the doctor my husband's address, and I never gave my family's address to him at all. Those who could help me were too far away in Turkey and Egypt; they only would be made very afraid. And, too, whenever I looked towards my children I told myself that I could not, would not, die. They were both too tiny to be sent into the care of other hands.

My husband had new work with a Tetuan journal and could not leave immediately. Also he did not believe, until his arrival in Lanjaron, that I was as severely ill as the doctor had claimed in writing to him. He knew well my exceptionally strong health: how, for example, through the past winter and early spring when we had been together in England, I had been able to bathe out-of-doors in icy rivers or tubs of rain-water, even when the long snow of that winter was deep on the ground. He knew also of my knowledge of herbal medicine, with which I had changed his own health from inferior to good. So when the bee in my dress stung me and the miller's wife foretold that Francisco would be at the mill within two days, it was quite prophetic, as he was not expected then at all.

Before Francisco arrived I was experiencing typhus delirium: when one raves and suffers daytime nightmares and there is no control over one's words and actions. Medical books tell that typhus patients often become very violent. I also was violent, but only against two persons – the miller's wife and the doctor. My violence towards the miller's wife was such that during my illness she always brought her son with her to protect her! I had no reason at all to be angry with her at that early time in the water-mill; perhaps I was foretelling events ahead.

I had every reason to be benevolent towards Patrocinio, for, with the help of a young woman from the town, she was caring for my children during my illness, and I, apart from taking them for walks during those times that I was mentally sane, and watching over their food, had no strength to do more for them. But even so, though the fever was great upon me, there were so many tasks that Patrocinio and the daily help left for me, that I was seldom able to lie quietly upon my bed before midnight came.

My anger towards the doctor was only a childish part of my illness. He wanted me to stay the day-long in my bed, and for me that was absolute defeat and an invitation to death to possess me, and I would not obey his commands. I was in the garden all the day. I bathed in the sun. And I bathed in the stream, many times, for as yet the water was almost unpolluted and came blue and cold from the sierra heights.

My craving for cold water was intense, both for drinking and bathing. Later, a doctor from Madrid told me that my instinct for cold-water bathing had very possibly helped to save me from death. Bathing the fever patients in cold water was an old Spanish cure for typhus, he said.

Often treatments have come instinctively to me. My brew of potato peelings, used internally and externally as part of a treatment against hard-pad, a high mortality disease in dogs, has proven greatly successful and has saved hundreds. During the time I had typhus, a letter came for me from my friend Adelita de Frederico in Mexico. She had copied out for me, from a very old herbal book of the Mexican Army, a cure for typhus: the basic element was potato peelings! I had not imagined that potatoes were known in Mexico so long ago – perhaps it was a wild form of that plant – but that was the cure that she copied out and sent to me, and it was the same treatment that I had given to the sick dogs.

Some fishermen of Torremolinos, beyond Malaga, told me that they remembered a typhus outbreak there in the nineteen-forties; those few men alone counted seven deaths among their relatives, all adults. They saved them by plunging them into baths of cold water; and their heads were shaved to check the inevitable hair-falling.

I treated myself by fasting from food, and drinking only lemon water sweetened with honey. Later I made use of garlic. For twenty-one days I abstained from all food. The miller's wife tried to urge me to eat, but my medical instinct and the will to live were strong, and I would not eat while the fever burnt in my blood. At the end of the three weeks there was no flesh on my body, I had become the skeleton form of the typhus phantom in his red cloak who kept such leering company at my bedside; but I was still alive and I could still walk quite strongly.

I was not aware of most of my strange actions during the typhus fever. The people at the mill, later, told me what I did. I think to relate all one's actions during delirium is as monotonous for other persons as the telling of one's dreams. But three things have a part in my record of Spanish typhus.

There was the pulling-down of my hair over my eyes. This I remember clearly. I used to pull down locks of hair and recite as dramatically as Lady Macbeth: "Black! Black! The plague! The plague!" The blackness of my hair used to frighten me then: it was the color of funeral pall. My hair obsession had good reason: I must have felt its pitiful dying. No one had told me, but one of the punishments of severe typhus is the loss of all one's hair. Both women and men have almost naked heads for three months or more while the new hair is growing. Scarves or wigs are worn. I wore a scarf! My hair, so thick that it was always an expense to me in broken combs, was scorched like the grass on the waterless parts of the Sierra Nevada, and it fell out in black handfuls, later, when the fever was ended.

I took midnight walks alone to the fountain on the land of the water-mill, and returned singing, holding a full jar of water. The path to the fountain is difficult even in daytime and countless people have fallen and become patients of the Sierra Nevada bone-setter, who is almost always sought at such times in preference to the town doctors.

The bone-setter in the region of the water-mill is a middle-aged man who works a high sierra farm. He is supposed to have the gift of God in his hands. I have seen several of his patients: all limbs were skillfully set and mended. The bone-setter dresses the limbs with a lotion of salt-and-vinegar, and then encases them in the orthodox plaster-bandage. But I never fell during those delirium walks; I only fell later when I was quite normal again, and one of the path-stones tilted beneath my feet. The arms of a tree caught me then and held me from the bad drop below, which had torn apart and painfully scarred the leg of Raphael, the miller's son, when he fell from that path.

Other sleep-walking turns took me to the cemetery. That cemetery of Lanjaron! I had disliked the place from before the birth of Luz. It was over-near to the water-mill. "Conveniently near," a person of Lanjaron had said to me when I was planning to leave the town for the mill. The white walls were so high the dead seemed to me to be imprisoned there. But what was more frightful to me was the great stone building which resembled a place for carrier pigeons, and in which place the dead were interred in small stone chambers. If my body had been interred there I would have haunted the lands of the near molino Gongoras.

The only cemetery that I have liked – and I have sad reason to visit many – was a Turkish one outside Smyrna. There my father is buried. There countless doves call their love one to another in the thickets of black cypress trees, and all around comes the music of sheep and goat bells. My father's tomb seemed peaceful. There was a strange thing about that tomb of marble. In a tiny crack grew a wild oat: golden and bold it waved to me in the winter wind. Like many Orientals my father was, unashamedly, a lover of women and in turn was greatly loved. I looked all around me at the other tombs and the grass stretches; not a wild oat to be seen, the seed set itself and grew on one tomb only. Oh, life is strange and sweet!

As I have written, I was little in my bed during typhus. The sunlight of the Spanish mountain made it possible for the children and me to be in the garden or on the mountain from sunrise to dusk. To be confined in one's bed when the sun is wonderful in the sky is undeserved punishment and I would not accept the doctor's commands. He was a good doctor for me because he was so pessimistic. His threats of "You will die! You will die!" were always a challenge. And he kept me well informed of my failing heart and pulse under the strain of the prolonged fever. He was a good friend to me in truth and I remember him gratefully.

Daily I used to drag myself up the rock steps and repose my thin, weak body against the strong one of an apricot tree, close by the upper mill-stream. There I used to read from a book which I had brought with me from England. I read always from the same book. I cannot tell why, but clearly it inspired me in my fight for survival. Perhaps it was the beauty of the book: perhaps because it told of another's pain and ultimate triumph — the crucifying of Christ. Two passages I read endlessly, from the *Revelations of Divine Love*, by the recluse nun, Julian of Norwich, were:

> "Also in this he [God] shewed me a little thing, the quantity of a hazel-nut, in the palm of my hand; and it was as round as a ball. I looked thereupon with eye of my understanding and thought: 'What may this be?' And it was generally answered thus: 'It is all that is made.' I marveled how it might last, for methought it might suddenly have fallen to naught for littleness. And I was answered in my understanding: 'It lasteth, and ever shall last for that God loveth it.' And so all things hath their Being by the love of God.
>
> "In this Little Thing I saw three properties. The first is that God made it; the second is that God loveth it; the third that God keepeth it."

The other passage is of the death of Christ: so tragic and painful and beautifully written.

> "I saw his sweet face as it were dry and bloodless with pale dying. And later, more pale, dead, languoring; and then turned more dead unto blue; and then more brown-blue, as the flesh turned more deeply dead. For his passion shewed to me most specially in his blessed face, and chiefly in his lips: there I saw these four colours, though it was afore fresh, ruddy, and liking to my sight. This was a sorrowful change to see, this deep dying. And also the nose clogged and dried, to my sight, and the sweet body was brown and black, all turned out of fair, lively color of itself, unto dry dying.
>
> "For that same time that our Lord and blessed Savior died upon the Rood, it was a dry, hard wind, and wondrous cold, as

to my sight, and what time the precious blood was bled out of the sweet body that might pass therefrom, yet there dwelled a moisture in the sweet flesh of Christ, as it was shewed.

"Bloodlessness and pain dried within; and blowing of wind and cold coming from without met together in the sweet body of Christ. And these four – twain without, and twain within – dried the flesh of Christ by process of time."

Dried the flesh by process of time! Week by week I could see my own flesh withering, from my head to my feet.

But my spirit remained well alive and the beauty of my daily companions in the mill garden, from the children to the bright grasses at my feet, inspired in me the will to survive the fever. The baby was always near by me, rosy and sweet in her Gypsy cradle of woven cane. And Rafik came and went, a sturdy, ruddy little lad, his nude body painted gold by the Spanish sun. Up and down the mill-path running or walking, went my little son, pulling his wooden toy cart laden with fallen quince blossom or pebbles and wrack from the stream.

And all around us the nightingales sang, singing best by day here on the Sierra Nevada. No mere one or two, but a company of lovely fluters in the quince trees and the bushes along the stream and above among the rocks. This I did not want to lose, would not lose. Nor the scent of the big red roses, handfuls of which Rafik pulled and brought to me, nor my love the wheat, which sang its song of the promised bread to come, food for the great grinding-stones of the mill, and food for my children and me; pale heads of the wheat turning to gold, green-ribboned with the streaming wind-blown leaves. These lovely things all close by me as I read from the nun's book.

Rafik used to play an endless game with me, hurtful because it was so true. It was a game of "going away," though in fact it was I who was likely to be going away on the long journey. And being a child's game it was ever played the same. Loading his cart with blossoms and wrack he would say:

"*Mi voy. Adios! Adios!*" (I go, good-bye).

"To where do you go?"

"Far! to Africa or Turkey, perhaps." Having association with those two countries, for North Africa was his birthplace, his choice was always so.

"Oh, that is very far, I shall cry!"

"I'll never come back again!" He would walk away.

"Then I shall cry more." I had to pretend to cry then; though sometimes real tears came indeed.

At that part of the game Rafik would come running back into my arms.

"Do not cry! I am back again!" Then, only a few minutes more, and the game would be performed once more.

"*Adios! Adios! Mi voy!*"

The flies plagued us in the garden, certainly a visitation from hell, but driving them away from the baby's cradle and from my body broke the typhus stupor which ever crept upon me in the horrible gray fog of its naming.

One of the most pleasant events of my mornings in the garden was a daily visit from my near neighbor – Asuncion Perez. She and her husband owned the river bathing-pool and were making colorful gardens there, though harassed by the destructive insects of the mountains which swarm to cultivated flowers. Always she brought me flowers: roses, and usually a magnificent geranium of flaring colors named "Gitana" (Gypsy). She told me the news of Spain and of the sierra. And above all she urged me to live.

"Fight this typhus. Fight. Fight," she would urge. "Children to pass their years without a mother's care and love, what a sad thing."

She herself was a wonderful mother, and had beautiful children. True Spanish beauties the elder girls. It was one of her daughters who had given me the thought of the name Luz for the baby. Luz, the famous shimmering light contrasted with shadow, on old buildings and sunburnt earth and mountains of Andalusia. The elder girls, Luz and

Ophelia, came to visit me often, also. Luz told me that she had dreamt that I would not die. She had seen me in her dream, very strong and sun-brown again, swimming in the pool. She promised that her dreams always came true.

My husband came to Lanjaron during the crisis of my illness. The typhus crisis is generally around the fourteenth day, when, if the patient is to recover, the fever abates, the brain clears and the languor diminishes. But around this time the strain upon the heart is so severe that death often results. The death-rate in epidemic typhus is given as from ten to one hundred percent, dependent on the form of the disease. For persons over fifty years of age it is fifty percent or more for most forms. It is significant that many of the leading research workers on typhus fever have themselves lost their lives to it.

In my case the crisis came at the end of one month of fever, and this seems to be quite general in the typhus of the Sierra Nevada area. Death came for me at the ending of that month – came very near. I could feel the cold clawing hands at my throat and heart, seeming indeed to be trying to pull my heart away out from my yet living body.

My spirit was away from my body then, floating around strangely, I think rather as the flights of a butterfly learning to use its newly come-by wings. As it flighted, my spirit seemed to take with it all the warmth from my flesh, leaving me cold and shriveled. My feet no longer seemed to feel the ground, it was as if I now ever walked over tall grass which swayed and bent beneath me. That my body was in a strange state was shown to me time and again when I sought to touch my children. My hands would reach out to touch them when in fact I was yet many yards away. My spirit had reached the children ahead of my body.

The morning came when I found with horror that I could not walk. I was defeated at last. Now I must stay in my bed, and lose the healing power of the sun and the water. Death would surely come. But I did walk! My husband was with me and he helped me, although he was very reluctant to defy the doctor's command that I must not leave my bed. With tremendous effort I reached the upper mill-stream and waded its length. The bright sunlit waters seemed to drive death away – only a few inches away certainly, but away!

In my room at the mill, throughout typhus I kept a bucket of fountain water near to my bedside. Countless times when the fever flared like flames upon me I would plunge my face, and then my arms, deep into that water, saying a prayer to the water such as once Saint Francis of Assisi had recited, but without his power of poetry. My prayer was, in intention, though often not fully spoken: "Oh, sweet fountain water! My shining friend, my silver love, pure, perfect, powerful healer and helper, save me!" I could not have endured without that water. As one further instance of my typhus delirium the miller's wife recalled to me. "I used to hear you talking to the bucket of water!"

That noon of the day when, almost, I could not walk, the doctor came in a taxi and took me away from the water-mill to a room in the town, closer to him. The doctor did not approve of the old dusty water-mill, and Francisco hated the place. It was unfortunate that my husband had come during the nesting time of the salamanders, which lived within the roof above my room. They rained earth and mortar dust upon his head!

I was used to such things, but he, who had lived most of his life in the clean town houses of Tetuan or Madrid, was not. He could never belong to the country life, and I, likewise, could not belong to the town. We warred much concerning this. He thought that it was madness on my part to choose to be alone in an old mill in Spain for the birth of our second child, and not with him in Tetuan.

He failed to find any of the beauty of the mill; he saw only its grime and lack of hygiene. But that was the fault of the present miller's wife. The mill itself was a rare thing, with its atmosphere of great age and great power, and the song of the wheat and maize, and the bread that came from the flours that its great stones made, all about it. And further, as I endeavored to explain to my husband, the children and I were seldom in the mill at all. We lived like Gypsies, either in the mill garden or out on the sierra. The day-long we lived thus, and even when night-time came we were almost outside, for the bed was in hand-reach of the door, and the door was never closed while I lived there – wide-open by day and night. Only during the day it was veiled with a curtain of netting (such as the fisher-folk of Portugal had taught me to use, although there we had used a true fishing-net) to keep out the flies.

My husband really blamed me for the fever, as doubtless will many more orthodox-minded people. But I am not the first traveler to have fever in Spain! And I was likely to be ill anyway because of the difficult pregnancy. Far better to have had the illness in the country where the mountain air and abundance of sunlight and fruits could restore the children and me to health.

The town room that the doctor had chosen for my use was clean and cool with a stone floor and a big window shaded by a Venetian blind – again for the reason of keeping out the flies – all quite typical of the Lanjaron houses. The big window fortunately faced a small garden, not the street, and I could hear faintly the stirring of the grape-vines over the trellis there. I could also hear my favorite birds, the swifts: their thin shrill screaming as they chased across the hot sky of mid-June; and they brought to me happy memories of my days in Granada with the Gypsies and with the Paris artist Georges Brunon, he painting the Gypsies and I writing about them.

The darkened room – caused by the necessary Venetian blind during the fly-hours of the day – proved most depressing to my mind and eyes. I missed the powerful song of the turning mill-wheel and grinding-stone. And above all, I missed my children. The awful pain of my separation from them came over me, and I knew that it would prove unbearable.

My son Rafik was as close to me as a faithful little hound. He knew all my moods and shared all with me. He was a nature-child and belonged to the Gypsy life. Gypsy children are bound close to their mothers until they are bodily and mentally strong enough to make independent lives of their own, and then they are given all the freedom that they desire. So it was with Rafik, and so it would be later: absolute freedom. But, meantime, it had meant careful education to get him to accept my absence for even a few hours. His father was almost a stranger to him, he was so much away, in the towns following his work as a journalist. Rafik warred with him.

I visioned, all too clearly, Rafik as he would be that long noon away from me. He would be running up and down the mill paths, calling for me, piteous-voiced as a golden plover calling and crying across the lonely places of the earth. I began to weep for him. Some more hours passed, and then I sent for the owner of the town-house and told her that she must take an urgent message to the doctor: That unless my son was brought to the town to be with me, I would not stay there but would return at once to the water-mill. I was not aware then of the great risk of typhus contagion – no one informed me. However, in the case of my children, they had been so much with me throughout the fever that if they were to take the disease it would already be incubating in their blood. And both yet seemed very well at that time.

Late that evening Francisco arrived with Rafik. The child's face, as I had rightly pictured, was swollen from hours of crying. He hurried to my bedside and took my hand.

"You have been away a long time," he said.

During the early days in the town room, the doctor was convinced that my condition was worsening. My heart was certainly greatly afflicted by the prolonged fever and my pulse seemed to have less power than a fluttering butterfly. But despite the adverse physical conditions with which doctors are always most concerned, I knew, with a tremendous surge of happiness, that I was getting better.

One important thing had happened to me since I had left the mill and had no tasks to do at all other than prepare meals for Rafik; my appetite for food had returned and after twenty-one days of absolute abstinence, I was eating again. At first taking little more food than that same butterfly; having to teach my body all over again to accept food, my jaws to grind, my unwilling throat to swallow, my stomach to digest. Moreover, I was eating real food, not the lifeless invalid diet which was habitual for Spanish typhus.

I refused the permitted dishes of bleached white rice powder and, instead, took foods which my body told me were needful to regain my strength: honey, and fruits of the sierra, and the typical and delicious white cheeses of the region, made from the milk of goats and ewes. I was also drinking quantities of water brought to me from the medicinal spring.

Soon came the time when I was able to read without difficulty again, and to write a little, in the feeble quavering style of a very old woman. But my hands strengthened daily, and I was writing normally within one week. I took many taxi rides to the roadway close by the water-mill, and staggered along the steep path to the mill door, where my baby was usually to be met with kicking in her basket and waving her hands at people.

My husband helped me on those difficult visits, for although it had been simple to learn again to eat and read and write, walking with normal strength and power came back to me very slowly. Finally the time came when I was able to do two things: walk, without help, to the water-mill, and swim in the pool. A short while after this, Francisco returned to Spanish Morocco to his work on the Tetuan journal.

Within a few days of his leaving, Rafik was clasped firmly in the arms of typhus fever. I was tormented at the thought of Rafik having now to experience the horror of typhus, perhaps as severe as I had known it. He was so little to know so cruel a disease.

I brought the doctor, Jiminez Moran, who had attended me, to Rafik's bedside, where the child lay in high fever; and the doctor confirmed my diagnosis.

"No injections," I said, "and no chemicals. I will care for him myself." I was given confidence to cure my child because of the numerous animals of all kinds which I had saved from death with the aid of herbal medicine.

Typhus was increasing in the district. I met people of the high sierra who were afraid to visit the town because so many of the people that they knew were typhus victims. In the case of Rafik and me, it was now certain that we had taken the disease from drinking polluted water. The upper mill-stream had been clean enough during the cold weather, when it was fed by the melting snows of the sierra, but later, and especially when the mill was grinding, it took up water from the river, where the town people came to wash their clothes, many of them doubtless having typhus in their homes at that time with the disease so general.

The miller's wife had assured me that the stream came directly from the sierra above, but later, some while after typhus, I followed the stream to its source, and saw how water both from the swimming-pool and the river leaked into it. Water has always been almost an obsession with me. I would not feed my body with dirty water, chlorinated and pumped through the pipes of the towns. Always, like the Arabs who almost worship the water of clean fountains and wells, I walked miles to such places for drinking water. I even collected such water for my dogs to drink. I think that perhaps I had foreknown that at some time in my life dirty water would bring death close to me.

Water plays such an important part in the body; how can true vibrant health be maintained on dirty and lifeless water? After I found the water polluted, I only used water from the fountain on the lands of the mill. It was a good distance from the mill to the fountain, and it took hours of my time walking to and fro to collect water for drinking, and for the children's baths, and again to wash the dishes there.

Even so, despite the fact that Rafik had drunk unclean water for months, I think that he would have remained immune from the typhus if he had not been out of my care for so long during my illness. Formerly he had had exceptional health. From the age of two months he had been traveling with me, and we had often been in parts of the world condemned as unhealthy. His good health was to help him in typhus as it had helped me.

When the doctor confirmed typhus, I asked him fearfully if he thought that my child would die. He then spoke words which rewarded me for all the care that I have taken to be rich – not in money, but in health. He said, "I will give you my opinion. You, yourself, have remarkable health. You are three times stronger than the normal person, otherwise you could never have survived the form of typhus which you developed so soon after the birth of your child. Your son is equally healthy; it will help him now as it has helped you. But you must know that typhus kills many children."

Kills many children! Soon after, I heard that my near neighbor, Maria, lost her son. He was around the same age as Rafik, and the two little boys had often played together. Her child died in four days she told me, crying: "Water! water!"

Rafik, too, cried for water; it was his chief delirium. But he did not die in four days. I will not write of his typhus. The memory of it is too painful and recent. And furthermore it would be a repetition of the description of my own illness. The fever, the delirium, the dysentery – the last rare in typhus, but typical of the form prevalent in the Sierra Nevada.

Rafik fasted voluntarily for seven days during the highest period of fever. He took only lemon water sweetened with honey, garlic water, and a fever drink which is much used in Andalusia: A strong tea of a mixture of three plants: leaves of eucalyptus (*Eucalyptus globulus*) and walnut (*Juglans nigra*), with the same measure of flowering stems and leaves of *altabacca* – a small yellow daisy-like flower used also to catch flies on its sticky and aromatic stems and leaves, bunches being hung from the ceiling on lengths of cord.

Another part of his treatment was a daily ride in his small open carriage. There were two reasons: a visit to the watermill to see Luz – from a distance always, so as not to expose her to further contagion; and to purchase a book or toy, both of which could be had for a few pence, and which fed his mind and strengthened him against the delirium. His presents, which he always chose himself, were arrayed on a chair by his bedside, and often they drew him out from a long spell of delirium.

A further important cure for his delirium seemed to be my tears. When I watched my very brave little boy fighting for his sanity, and knew that he was being hugged to the bony breast of the red-cloaked fiend, typhus, my tears would rain from my eyes in storms and fall upon the strained face of the child–and always he would come back to sanity and knowledge of my presence, and say in Spanish "Don't cry, mamma." That lovely Spanish word, to weep, *llorar*.

The concern of the people of Lanjaron for Rafik and me, and the baby, was heartening. Gifts of fruit came to us from gardens and *cortijos* (small ranches); an abundance of love was expressed in bunches of summer flowers. The Gypsies brought us medicinal herbs. My opinion concerning the Spanish people, formed over several years, is that they are very kind and compassionate and possess ample and generous hearts, especially the women, and most of all the Gypsies and the true peasants. The men are sometimes rather vain and likewise selfish; especially the very handsome ones. But I love them – selfish handsome men and all!

This concern for Rafik and me during the typhus affliction was half a year before the news of the hydrogen bomb menace came to us. Then, the life of one woman and one child – both nearly strangers to them – seemed to possess much importance. Now that we are all threatened with wholesale annihilation of the human race, individual lives may not matter, outside the immediate family.

But I have absolute faith – formed out of my own life experiences, the misfortunes and the miracles, many miracles, that I have seen – that every individual being, from a flower to a child, is of concern to the Creator of life. Other-

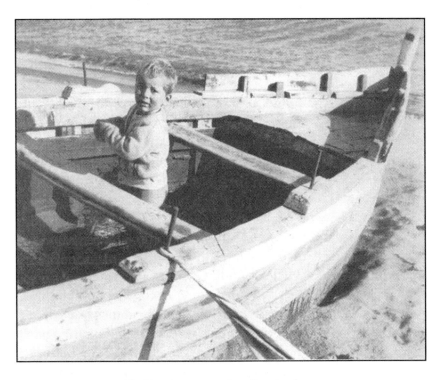

Rafik, strong again after typhus.
Photo by Marcus Hohenthal

wise, our prayers would not have been answered, and we would have died of the typhus. All the culture that man has created in the better hours cannot be blown into nothingness by atomic bombs. Whatever the future may bring, horror or glory, my belief will remain with me, and I will teach it to my children. We have made a small beginning already by not accepting the deaths of animals – either for food or for the sake of medicine.

In times of uncertainty I can always recall the words of the nun Julian of Norwich, whose writings held my mind during the typhus, especially as to the little hazel-nut, which might have dissolved into nothing for its very littleness, but which "lasteth and ever shall last for that God loveth it." There is true power in the nun's words because of their sweet simplicity. They are such an important contrast to the rantings of intemperate statesmen who are bloated with power, overrich, and living unnaturally.

Rafik soon conquered the typhus and regained his former good health. The deep coral tints were beautiful on his face as before, and, best of all, he was able to walk again without falling. That had been most painful to witness – a child unable to walk, for the great weakness had replaced his former magnificent strength. Sad enough when adults cannot walk, but far, far, sadder for children, their pleasure being to run and romp. Rafik did not romp again for a long time, but he walked.

The mountain gave me the herbs I needed to cure Rafik, for no chemical medicine from the pharmacy came near him during his illness. The abundant sunlight and the cool fresh air of the mountain nights likewise helped. The polluted water which had brought disease to the child and me was no fault of the mountain, but of humans who, in stupidity and ignorance, befoul precious things, especially the waters of the earth which should be kept clean as a shrine and worshipped. Therefore I and my children continued to love the mountain.

Chapter Five

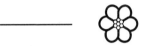

Sierra Nevada Processions

From my first days on the Sierra Nevada and onwards, there was an endless succession of religious processions. They were the chief entertainment for the family of the molino Gongoras, and big bunches of the flowers from the mill garden enhanced them; especially those fair night-scented phlox-like blossoms, flower of San Pedro (*Hesperis matronalis*).

Most of the processions, to my eyes, were garish and almost vulgar, with the firing of rockets tearing one's ears. In a country so rich in flowers, especially the wild ones of the mountain, it was a sadness to me that most of the floral decorations used in the processions were artificial.

One of the early processions of the Sierra Nevada, I loved. That was the celebration of the day of Saint Marco: the blessing of bread and the animals of the sierra.

The statue of Saint Marco was brought out from Lanjaron church. The figure was swart-faced and dark-haired, garlanded with flowers (artificial!) and necklaced and braceleted with little rings of bread called the *roccas* of Saint Marco. More strings of the little breads hung from the shoulders, and a crown of one large *rocca* was around the head. The children of the town also wore tiny *roccas* fastened like brooches to their jackets or dresses, baked by their mothers or purchased from the bakeries who in turn had helped to decorate the statue of their patron saint.

Far along the road both to and away from the church, all those animals which are such an important part of the life of the Sierra Nevada, were herded or tethered for the saint's blessings. In large numbers there were horses, mules and donkeys, cows, goats, sheep and shepherd dogs, hens and pigs, pigeons; and close in the wake of the statue, teeming herds and flocks of cows, goats and sheep, the collar bells of the two last animals glinting in the bright sunlight and swinging and ringing. With such a rush of swift feet and the scent of rosemary and olive-wood and the sweet new grasses and herbs of the sierra, the animals passed by.

The statue of Saint Marco was carried by six Gypsies. The Gypsies and the church are not generally associated, but in Spain there is often close attachment. I think that the Gypsies were favored with the bearing of Saint Marco, because of their important part in the animal life of the Sierra Nevada. A big proportion of the animal trading was in their hands, especially the transport animals: horses, mules and donkeys. They also sheared and clipped the animals for the peasants and townsmen during the hot spring and summer months, and are expert in this.

Sadly, they slaughtered them, too. The meat trade of Lanjaron was almost entirely in Gypsy hands. The Gypsies bought the animals young, herded them on the mountain and then would slay them to supply the big demand for meat during the five months that visitors crowd to the Lanjaron area of the sierra to drink the medicinal waters of the famous spring. It was a very general sight to see Gypsy youths and men herding huge flocks of goats, often numbering over one hundred, and bulls also; they are never chained, but running loose on the mountains and controlled merely by a long cane.

The Gypsies, with their especial inherent powers with animals, were most successful herdsmen. Also they well knew the true value of all livestock, and if they had any friendship with a non-Gypsy they were the best people from whom to purchase an animal, for they bought cheap and they sold cheap. The goat at the water-mill, who later played an important part in my life there, was a Gypsy goat; she had been reared by and bought from the Romanies.

The demeanor of the Gypsy men carrying the statue of the saint – all of them handsome, with their shaggy black hair and swart, lean faces – was not very holy! They flashed their eyes and laughed with their thin dark-lipped mouths at the Gypsy girls and women who were grouped in the street. The day of Saint Marco, similar to the day of Saint Juan, later, was a special day for the Gypsies.

As the statue of Saint Marco passed away down the street, there came great clamor from the animals and the children; and the children then promptly began to nibble at the toy bread rings, their *roccas* of Saint Marco. I loved all of that procession, from the thronging animals to the unholy statue bearers, and I was sad, not relieved, as with all the other previous processions, when it came to an end.

The later procession of *Corpus Christi* was sheer loveliness, perhaps because it passed by at night-time, in the lamplight: it had the quality of a dream. I have seen many processions in different parts of the world, but no one of them stirred my heart like the *Corpus Christi* procession of the Sierra Nevada, which brought tears; I think because it was so simple and divine, with a passion for Christ. And, furthermore it was so personally linked with the recovery of my child and myself from typhus. He, at the time of the procession, was sleeping quietly in his bed, free at last from the terrible fever and delirium. The tears came because we were both in life and I was seeing much beauty.

Corpus Christi celebration in Spain is purely a manifestation of love for Christ – *El Señor* – and faith in Him and the Church of which He is the heart. And June is a happy time in which to adore.

So, at eight o'clock on that June night, the Lanjaron *Corpus Christi* procession passed along the main street, with the swifts still present in the sky, screaming and flighting in dark arrow sallies across the purple-blue.

That one center street of the town was much decorated by the house-owners: hung with garlands of flowers, mostly carnations and madonna lilies and the wild golden butterfly broom from the lower slopes of the mountain. Every house balcony was draped either with the famous embroidered shawls of Spain or cloths of hand-worked lace, delicate as gypsophila flowers, or with fine carpets and rugs. The house where I stayed during the last days of my typhus had an ugly pink tablecloth decorating the balcony! But they were such good people the cloth seemed to me to be quite lovely that night.

Heading the procession came little boys in white satin suits carrying sheaves of madonna lilies and prayer books. They were the rich children of the district, or sons of the town merchants. Behind them followed the peasant lads, with flesh all copper-glow from the sierra sun. Goat- and sheep-herds mostly, those little brown lads, clad in corduroy trousers and sun-faded and patched shirts. They carried only candles. The light from their flickering flames moved like fireflies about the dark solemn faces.

Then marched the town band, wearing uniforms of gray. For hours, from midnight until the dawn of the day of *Corpus Christi*, they had played their quite sad and haunting old tunes of Spain up and down the village street. Their music was then superseded by the truly unearthly flamenco-like chanting of the *saetas* whose passionate religious chorusing I shall always associate in Spain with the march of the *penitentes*, those strange tall-hooded and masked Ku-Klux-Klan-like figures, ghostly in their black or white garb, boys as well as men parading.

Then, loveliest of all to my eyes, came the little girls, mostly of First Communion, wearing their bride-like church dresses and head-veils of white, the shortest children first and then going upwards to the tallest ones in the rear. The little girls did not walk, they skipped and tossed like the wild white marguerites breeze-blown on the lower slopes of the mountain. Each child carried a small basket heaped with dried flowers; roses mostly, but also others of the lovely scented flowers, white and purple violets, lilies-of-the-valley, carnations, jasmine. Two of the little girls, the tall ones, were quarreling as they walked by me. One of them had snatched flowers from the basket of the other, and they were pulling at one another's long black ringlets (in which style most of the children wore their hair that night of the procession). Order among the girls was being kept by a child not more than ten years old. She hustled around keeping the little white dolls in straight rows, and she reprimanded the quarreling pair and had them walk a goodly distance apart. So much authority coming from a small child was remarkable.

In the rear of the girl children walked the important men of the town: the big merchants and some little merchants, doctors and men in retirement, and all alongside the procession walked black-gowned women carrying lighted candles: the Sisters of Jesus. To be a Sister of Jesus a small sum of money must be paid to the church every year, and special church duties fulfilled.

Then, slow of pace, solemn, the very essence of the Catholic Church, came the priests, holding torches and swinging hand-braziers of burning incense, scenting the street with rich – and always mysterious – perfume. Their tonsured heads were lit by the flare of the torches ahead, their long black robes flapped like the wings of ravens, and over their shoulders lay short capes of white lace, of the same fine and beautiful hand-work as seen in the lace cloths decorating the house balconies. In the center of the group of priests was the High Priest of the church, more beautifully adorned than the others, the representative of the Christ. He attracted to himself a most sweet rite: the strewing of flowers.

For again and again, two by two, the smallest of the little girls broke from their group and, running to the Head Priest, strewed their flowers, not at his feet but upwards towards his heart. Throughout the marching of the procession the girl children emptied their baskets of blossoms upon the representative of *El Señor*.

My baby Luz was in that procession of *Corpus Christi*, dressed in her best white dress embroidered with swallows. She was carried in the arms of the miller's wife. I did not see her. I would not have approved of Luz being out in the cold mountain air so late, but others saw her pass by.

The more I see of the pageantry of the Catholic church the more I admire. It is a pity that the warlike firing of rockets has become a part of the pageantry, but for the rest there is only beauty. Above all the church belongs very much to the people, to the poor equally with the rich: The very poor bring their offerings of wild flowers. I well remember in Mexico the happiness of a Catholic church where Mexicans and half-caste Spanish-Indians were celebrating the midnight mass on a Christmas eve. The people had journeyed long distances to the church from the small ranches and shacks of that part of the Baja California peninsula. They had journeyed mostly on horses and donkeys, accompanied by their ranch dogs.

And the lean shaggy dogs were allowed entry into the church and lay at the feet of their masters. Stocky, swarthy women suckled their babies, the children ate candy and maize cakes, and the air was thick with the scent of garlic breath and hot unwashed bodies. The singing was fervent and heartfelt and an atmosphere of real happiness prevailed. When I spoke with the priest about the dogs in the church, he smiled and said: "Why not! It is their church. The horses and donkeys could have entry also if the door were bigger. Bless them!"

Personally I have no church. As a child I attended, with my parents, the synagogue of the Sefardi Spanish and Portuguese Jews, but now, in adulthood, I take the beauty of them all: church, synagogue, mosque. And the Sierra Nevada procession of *Corpus Christi* was a memorable part of the search for beauty of all kinds.

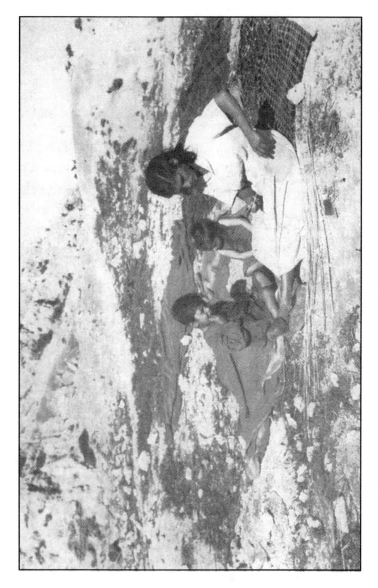

Gypsy basket maker; the beginning of a basket. Photo by Marcus Hohenthal

Chapter Six

The Gypsies

In almost every town and village of the Sierra Nevada there are Gypsies, and in the environs of Lanjaron there are very many. The Sierra Nevada is ideal for Gypsy life: there is space and light, streams and natural fountains, and almost always the sun. Away from the small farms and the mule paths the land is wild and savage and there is an abundance of wild fruits and edible plants, also many unfenced cultivated crops on which the Gypsies, unfortunately, prey. I know of no Gypsy around Lanjaron who cultivates much land, as they do in other parts of the sierra and in many parts of Portugal, where the Gypsies quite often own sizeable farms where they raise fine horses and mules. Many of the Sierra Nevada Gypsies are nomads, traveling the sierra with animals or attending the principal fairs of Spain, of which there are very many.

The Lanjaron Gypsies herd animals on the sierra and gather willows and river cane and reeds and many other shrubs and plants for their chief work, which is basket-making. The butcher trade is also in their hands, and they hawk clothing and lengths of cloth, mostly cloth, of which the Spanish women buy very much, attracted by its customary cheapness. They are rarely nomad and mostly live crowded in the twin Gypsy quarters of the town. The big quarter, Cueta, behind the town and facing the river – into which pours all the filth of the latrines – and the little one close to the cemetery and the water-mill.

Although Lanjaron belongs to Granada and shares the same mountains of the Nevada, the Gypsies of the two places are so different they seem like people from entirely different lands, as though they were months of journeying away, not the mere two-hour bus ride between Granada and Lanjaron. The Lanjaron Gypsies are mostly serious and industrious, with the exception of fiesta days, whereas the Granada ones are mostly frivolous and occupied with catch-penny trades, apart from those who perform the more arduous work of professional dancing, singing and music.

The serious work of the Lanjaron Gypsies is weaving with willow, cane, and various other plants most beautiful articles, from baskets to babies' cradles. My baby Luz passed her infant days in a Gypsy cradle, light and supple and yet very warm. Eventually I took it to England with me. But I had to save it first from bed bugs, very common invaders of wicker-work in southern Spain. For sentimental reasons I refused to abandon that cradle. I drowned the bugs by sea-bathing it over one hundred times.

In the Gypsy quarter almost every doorstep was occupied with dark-skinned lean-bodied people weaving baskets and cradles or chair seats. They sang as they worked: a deep throbbing chant, something like the famous chorusing of the Gypsy copper-beaters around Granada and elsewhere.

The miller's two sons went away many days on their donkey and brought back great bundles of willow and cane. The willow they stripped and later sold to the Gypsies, who, they told me, bought for almost nothing and sold their wares later very dearly. But as very few of the Sierra Nevada peasants could weave baskets, they almost all bought in quantities from the Gypsies and at the Romany prices. Every year a party of Gypsy weavers came to the water-mill of Gongoras for a day or more and wove baskets for the family Lopez, from the *mimbre* that the miller's sons had collected and peeled. They came in early April the year that I was there, and wove in one day many beautiful baskets.

I formed a friendship with that family Heredia; and I asked them to weave the baby's cradle, for she was soon to be born.

Later the daughter, Maria, came to help me when I sickened with typhus fever. She was sweet with the baby Luz, crooning Gypsy songs to her and never tiring of holding the baby in her arms. Then Maria too developed typhus and went away. I do not think that she took typhus from me at the water-mill for she had the lesser form, quite unlike the type that I suffered. She came back again to me when she was better; I did not need help then for I was strong again myself, but she came for love of Luz and to wash her one dress in the mill-stream and dry it in the sun.

When I think of the garden by the upper mill-stream, one of my chief memories is of Maria sitting there, slim and ivory-skinned − for she was of the basket-weavers and did not know the sun, always sitting on her family's doorstep on the shady side of the street − clad only in a ragged black slip, waiting for her one dress to dry. I have few enough dresses myself, as such things nowadays have not the former importance for me, and like the Gypsies I like old and ragged ones which seem to hold an especial friendliness for one's body − but I intend to give Maria a dress or two.

Below the water-mill and within hearing of the mill, was a public washing-trough, where the Gypsies from the nearby quarter, and also women of the town, came daily to wash their linen in the water which came down from the mill. The children of the non-Gypsies sat quietly by the trough as their mothers did their washing, but the Gypsy children played like goat kids upon the rocks, leaping and prancing and chasing. They made castanet music from two pebbles, showing an excellent sense of rhythm. I recall seeing by the washing trough two young Gypsy children, brother and sister, weaving a nest most skillfully from the fallen golden wand-blossom of the chestnut trees, which were then abundant on the sierra for miles distant. The bird they were helping – a young swallow from the water-mill – would die in a day, surely; but I did not tell the children this.

There was another washing place much used by the Gypsy women, a deep pool in the river, almost facing the mill. It was there that they sang as they washed their clothes or washed articles for other people. During the season of the Lanjaron medicinal springs they would often dress themselves up in the clothes of the rich tourists which they were to wash, and they would then masquerade. The pajamas which such people wore for sleeping always amused the Gypsies for they seldom possess night-clothes, generally sleeping either in their clothes of the day or in healthy nakedness.

Immediately after my typhus fever, though I was scarcely able to walk, I went often to the mill to see my baby and sometimes further, to bathe in the pool. Once, I fell there, in the then-shallow river, and I was too weak to get away from the slippery rocks. It was a young Gypsy woman who lifted me out, and then washed the mud from my skirt and from the two bathing towels which I was carrying.

Dolores Carmona was my favorite Gypsy in Lanjaron; from that day I came to know her well. Very lovely, she reminded me of a fritillary flower, for she was fair and freckled, slim and lithe and yet exotic. She had fame among the Lanjaron Gypsies for her singing and dancing. It was a true sadness for all of us when she ran away to Valencia with a lover. "Old and ugly and not even rich," was the description of the lover given by the Lanjaron Gypsies. They were angry because she had chosen a non-Gypsy for her romance. I found the passion for their race, their "kawlo rat" blood, very strong among the Lanjaron Romanies.

The day of Saint Juan is a special day for the Sierra Nevada Gypsies; Saint Juan himself was a shepherd before he left the mountains to be with Christ. A very large proportion of the Gypsy population possessed the name of Juan (or Juanita for the girls). Around Lanjaron, on that saint's day, it was traditional for the Romanies to bathe their faces in the River Husagre soon after dawn, to wear their best clothes, and throughout the night, to hold fiesta. One of the traditional places for this dancing was the court of the watermill, perhaps because of its nearness to the river.

All my life I shall remember the night of Saint Juan, for that was one of the two successive nights when Luz was apparently dying.

This is not to be a book about my family. It is about Spanish mountain life, but where the life comes into my family it is not out of place that I should write about my children.

On that night of Saint Juan, a few Gypsies came to the mill for the customary dancing and singing, about twenty in all. Not many of the Lanjaron Gypsies have any liking for the present miller's wife, and therefore they held their fiesta elsewhere. In all, about twenty adults came; most of them had children who danced also, with the exception of the very young.

I could see that Luz was very ill. Her six weeks in the care of Patrocinio had exhausted all of her natural babyhood health; she was as a little sprig of the plant of life, without any leaves or flowers at all. Hour by hour, every day since my return to the water-mill, I had worked to remove the ill-health which had come to my baby and replace ill with good; but I often felt, terror-stricken, that it was too late. On the night of Saint Juan, my frightened eyes showed me clearly that my previous doubts were realized.

The Gypsy dancing and singing commenced as soon as the first stars appeared; I could hear the celebrating in my room. We had all been looking forward to that night; but now, for me, all had become dark and drear. The celebrating below only overwhelmed me with bitterness and despair, so much so that I finally closed my door to keep from my ears the sound of other people's happiness. I knew positively that if I should lose Luz I should never know true happiness again. In the weeks of struggle to save my baby from her unfortunate fostering, she had become very dear to me: she was so loving and grateful and brave in her pain.

Dr. Jiminez Moran, who came several times to see Luz, said rightly that he felt sadder when a young person died than when an adult did. And I felt this utter sadness for my baby: to have been born into the world, known pain, and then banished, having seen scarcely anything of the earth's endless beauty. Never to have understood how much she was loved by her mother and loyal little brother; not to have romped in meadows and bathed in streams; nor seen her pretty face in a mirror. Oh, a thousand things. Chrysalis never to have become butterfly. What a pity! How cruel! Cruel!

Many and many a time there came the rapping of Gypsy hands upon my closed door, and their voices calling for me to come below and be with them. Every time Rafik pleaded tearfully that we should do so; since babyhood he had been much with the Gypsies and he loved them. Finally there came the old Gypsy of Lanjaron whom the others called *El Antigua* (The Old One). She said that the Gypsies were very sad that I was not with them on their special night, that they understood my reason for staying away and closing my door, but they wanted to dance and sing for me, to make the baby well again.

I could not resist such pleading. I put on a bright dress and took the two children below to the courtyard. I knew that the Gypsies expected the bright dress; they might be in rags themselves but they liked their guests to be "dressed-up."

We were given a sincere welcome by all and the dancing became wilder and the singing louder. And one by one the Gypsies came to wish better health for Luz. But I could see in their dark eyes the same fears for her which possessed me. Then, when I had been at the fiesta an hour, I heard a Gypsy woman sitting nearby tell her husband that she could not bear to remain in sight of the baby and watch her dying, that she had to sit further away. Then I could hold back no more my increasing fears and grief, and I went back to my room. Rafik stayed with the Gypsies, and his powerful voice came to me in imitative calls of Gypsy songs.

Oh, that flamenco singing of the night of Saint Juan! The age-old passion and frenzy and grief of the Moors within, and without, the howl of the winds from barren Spanish plains and mountain heights, the croon of mountain streams and pouring fountains. And the beat of the tambours: tambours for war and tambours for love.

Not one of the family of the water-mill came to visit Luz that night. Patrocinio, who had mothered my baby for nearly two months and must know that she was passing from life, was too busy selling wine and soda drinks to the people making fiesta. Alone, Señor Jose came faithfully to bring me water from the fountain, and to carry Rafik – who was overcome by sleep while enjoying the revelry – from the courtyard to his bed.

The old woman, *El Antigua*, came around midnight with her daughter, declaring that I should not be alone at such a time. The daughter, Pura, told me that her own child, Carmen, had been abandoned by the doctors but had recovered. I knew Carmen well and admired her for her vivacious nature and the brightness of her singing as she washed clothes in the river. Pura said that she would send for Carmen to confirm this and thus to give me faith.

Carmen came later, around one in the morning, and confirmed her mother's account of her near death, and told me that she had a premonition that Luz, also, would not die. Then the Gypsies left my room for I told them that I would not steal their sleep; I knew they all had work to do on the morrow; and furthermore Rafik was company. No matter that he was asleep; my little lad was company and also inspiration.

I was inspired! The baby had much pain from the weeks of faulty diet and improper care. Her pain had kept her from sleep for a day and a night. I suddenly bethought myself of a group of white opium poppies which I had seen in flower in the upper mill garden. Those poppies were certainly part of that night of Saint Juan, for they died away then and never came again, while I was at the water-mill, and I don't remember seeing them in flower before. I made a brew of the gray-green heads from which the white petals had fallen, and gave Luz sips of that medicine mixed with honey. This very quickly lessened the pain, but I knew that it was a desperate and dangerous medicine, for it made yet colder her

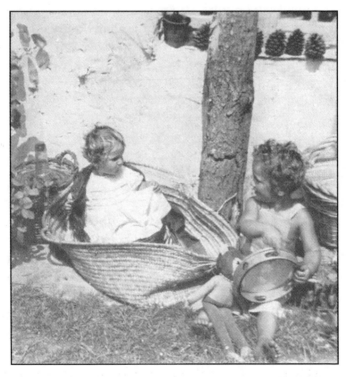

Fiesta! Luz in her Gypsy cradle commences a Spanish dance.
Photo by the author

already over-cold body. But she did not die. That night of Saint Juan she was as cold and white as the opium poppies themselves, but she did not die.

The next day she remained the same, but with the night, she suddenly worsened. That was the crisis. I remembered that the Gypsy Carmen had not died and she had promised that Luz would not die. I sent for the doctor, wanting him to check her heart and respiration; and then the great wound came to me.

He said, in quick Spanish to Patrocinio, that Luz was dying and she must be prepared for this.

"*Cuando?*" (When?), I asked of him, and his face paled at my having heard his words and at the way my voice sounded.

"Any hour," he replied, lowering his eyes.

I will not write about the symptoms of life's ending which I saw upon my baby. But well I recall my quite childish words.

"I will not let her die!" I cried. I held Luz against my heart. I was like a child about to be deprived of a doll which she loved. I would not give her up to anyone; I would not.

Dr. Moran said that Luz must have penicillin injections. That was a great test for me. I am absolutely opposed to injections. Always they are a shock to the body and do much damage to the nerves. Any medicine of any value at all should be able to be taken into the body by the mouth: the natural place for medicines. But penicillin is at least plant-like and was not evolved from cruel experiments on animals, therefore I agreed to that medical treatment.

I also continued with the opium medicine, and a further brew of dill seed with much honey, to save the tiny laboring heart. The following day a different doctor suggested tissue infusions of the medicinal water of Lanjaron. To this, also, I agreed. Which part of the treatment saved the baby, I do not know. But she lived!

As with Rafik, so Luz's illness also passed. The dawn came, the swallows twittered, and my baby lay safe in her

Gypsy cradle. Personally, if I were to choose the treatments which I think most helped her, indeed saved her, it would be the three days' fasting from all food, combined with an external treatment which I had learned a summer ago from Portuguese fisher-women, of massaging the stomach area time and again, night and day, with hot olive oil and pounded aniseed. To me, these were the most important remedies of all the many which kept my baby from death. And further: Fervent prayer, and the good wishes of the Gypsies who came to Luz that night of Saint Juan and thereafter, surely saved her.

When the crisis was one week ended, Rosario Heredia, an eighteen-year-old Gypsy girl, came to offer her milk for Luz. She had a son, Juan, born close to the same time as my baby. I remember the birth of Juan: I used to send gifts of goat's milk for Rosario, who had been rather weak at that time. Luz fed at the gypsy's breast for nearly one month, until Rosario's milk became insufficient. It seemed to me a Gauguin picture: Rosario with Luz at her tawny breast, red geraniums in her charcoal-black Gypsy hair, her short strong body squatting – Native American-fashion – upon the green turf by the mill-stream in the shade of the quince trees, which were at that time decorated with their pale green-yellow lamps of fruit. Rosario sang to Luz, songs almost as endless as the chant of the coursing mill-stream, Gypsy songs and other songs of Spain. The one which Luz seemed to like best and which Rosario sang most often was a sweet and simple thing:

> *Oh green eyes! Green as the eyes of cows,*
> *Green as the first tassels of the wheat*
> *And green as the early lemons.*

Rosario had none of the sweetness and kindliness of my other Gypsy friend Maria of the basket-makers. Rosario was tawny and fierce as a tiger; perhaps she reminded me of a tiger because she preyed on others. She was an incurable

monger – a Gypsy word for beggar. She came from a mongering family. From her equally tiger-like but very tall mother
to her youngest sister, all pestered me for money and articles
which I was often in need of for my own family. I never
gave to that begging family one peseta. But to Rosario I gave
a new green apron, and a green and white skirt which she
chose, of exactly the same material and pattern as my own.
We looked like sisters when we went into the town together!
And I gave her also a gaudy scarf such as the Gypsies love,
for her milk had greatly helped my baby.

I found Rosario intelligent and humorous and I loved
to talk with her because, as with most mongerers, her speech
was fanciful. For instance, she told me once of another water-mill which was to be rented. She described a paradise!
An old mill set in a beautifully kept garden, filled with roses
and lilies and fruit trees: endless clean water all around and
a river deep enough for swimming. At that time the mill-
streams of Gongoras were being polluted, the garden was
barren and dry, and I wanted to leave.

One very hot morning I went with Rosario to see the
other water-mill. It was all mirthful. The mill was almost
derelict. The one room suggested for the use of my family
was without roof or door and teemed with ants. But most important of all was the state of the water: it came polluted by
excreta from the town above, and the river nearby not only
was of such shallowness that only in very few places did it
reach one's knees, and furthermore, it stank from the dirty
waters which fed it. The water-mill of Gongoras was at least
above the town and away from it, not below, as with this mill!

Rosario's milk was succeeded by a Gypsy goat who gave
my Luz her milk. Luz, being Andalusian born, followed the
custom of that region and fed direct from the goat's udder.
Thus, despite the great heat of the summer, her drinks of
milk were always sweet and fresh. The number of Sierra Nevada children who have been fed by goats, sheep, and even

cows and donkeys, is very great, although it is becoming more rare nowadays. It is also frequent custom among the Arabs and was very probably taught to the Spanish by the Moors.

All around me were people who, as babies, had been fed directly by milk animals. The miller himself had been reared on a goat; the mother of Señora Perez, likewise, and Sebastian, one of the strongest Gypsies of Lanjaron and about the best swimmer there, all were goat-reared. The big-built, popular Pepe, proprietor of the Cafe Suizo, had fed from a donkey; and the milk of asses is said, on the Sierra Nevada, to be the most healthful of all for children. But I was content for a goat to foster my baby, for I love that race of animals.

So many people have been goat-reared on the sierra, that there are, understandably, many beliefs concerning this. They say that children fostered by goats grow up into noble adults. Certainly Señor José was a very good and forthright man; and Señora Rafaelita – of the swimming-pool – most noble and a lover of nature, hence the fine flowers that she grew in the Lanjaron river garden.

The people said also, that when a person who has fed from a goat dies, the goat, no matter how strong and how youthful, dies also. There were also tales told of goats who stood over the cradles of babes whom they were fostering, so that the babes could drink their milk whenever the cries of hunger came to their listening ears.

Luz's Gypsy goat, black and tall and shaggy, topaz-eyed, never stood over the cradle, but did often come to the baby to nuzzle her, and did know the hours of her feeding and would alone mount the steep steps to the upper mill-stream and there seek out Luz wherever her cradle was situated.

There is an Andalusian legend concerning a prince who was suckled by a goat, and which tells also of the origin of the Milky Way. This prince was a son of a "King of the Orient" (perhaps a Gypsy) who long ago had dwelt on a high mountain which pierced the skies. Soon after the birth of the prince, the queen fell ill and her milk failed altogether. She was too jealous to let another woman foster her son, and instead a beautiful white goat was brought into the palace apartments. The baby prince fed from the goat's udder and grew so strong that the king would take the child with him when he went hunting in his forests. One day, the prince fell unnoticed from his father's saddle, and was lost in a dense part of a forest. The white goat wept like a woman and refused to allow anyone to take her milk from her. Days went by, and on the third, the frenzied goat broke free from the chains which held her and ran from the palace to search for the little prince, whom no one had been able to find. Her udder was bursting with the milk that she had held so long for the child she loved, and as she ran, the milk dripped from her udder, leaving a white trail.

Eventually the goat found the prince, near to death from days of starvation; she fed him lovingly. The king tracked the goat by the trail of milk she left, and thus met with his son alive and well, saved by the faithful goat. The king opened his wallet and strewed handfuls of diamonds upon the goat, and did thus all the way back to the palace. And in this wise there came into being across the sky The Milky Way: the white trail of the goat's milk, and the strewn diamonds which turned into stars.

I must tell of the Gypsy caravan which passed through Lanjaron before the Holy Week celebrations. For although they did not belong to Lanjaron they belonged to the Sierra Nevada.

This family were the most typical nomad Gypsies whom I had met during all of my travels, with the exception of Turkish Romanies who were yet wilder and more true to the ancient type of nomad. Those sierra Gypsies were traveling from village to village on the mountain, making and selling artificial flowers, primarily for the Holy Week festivals; the men also trading mules and donkeys, of which animals they had long strings traveling along with them.

Spanish Mountain Life

I was walking with some people from Lanjaron at the time of the Gypsies' arrival, and they warned me not to talk with such. They said, "Our own *gitanos* are bad enough, but these are the kind who knock down people in robbery and then move on. No one knows from where they have come and to where they are going. And how black they are!"

Black they were indeed! And ugly! This ugliest pack of Gypsies did not seem so much human, but rather wolves dressed up in gaudy clothes. They were dark and lean, with slitty, glittering eyes, and long yellow teeth. The men mostly possessed thick black moustaches with curled-up ends, and wore wide-brimmed greasy hats, and their slitty eyes laughed at me from out the shadows of the hat brims. Those Gypsies did not seem part of this present world, but rather as if they had come out from the Spanish past, the old life of the Sierra Nevada, the savage past before the present taming. Not to stay and talk with such wonderful people was absurd, so I stayed alone with Rafik, and the others walked on.

I bought three of their red paper roses and put them in my hair, and that pleased the Gypsies and the women made a place for me to sit with them and watch them as they worked. Between times I bartered with the men for a tiger-striped greyhound with yellow eyes, which they possessed. They asked me for twenty duros for the greyhound, less than an English pound note, and the dog was worth five pounds or more. But I had no time to give to the care of a dog with my baby then soon to be born, and moreover, I know greyhounds, and that dog was of powerful personality and intelligence. He would not like my present fettered life, and doubtless at the first chance he would be away: as swift and as not-to-be-caught as a star falling, seeking out his Gypsy masters again. I told the men this, and they laughed and said "maybe."

The women were true artists at their flower-making. They had pots of paint, and they painted the little clay pots all the colors of the gaudy Orient, and into those pots they placed their paper flowers on wire stems wound around with pale green paper, the wire stems supported in wet earth mixed with clay. Their flowers were roses, yellow and red poppies, carnations of many hues, and the holy lilies. In each stiff white corolla of the lilies they painted yellow rays, and soon they had me too painting in the rays for them. I was amused with the paint-brush as in childhood days, and Rafik too was knowing joyous hours, for along with the Gypsy children, he was busy handing earth into the little rainbow pots.

It was one of my happiest times on the Sierra Nevada, and for memory of our morning together, the Gypsies gave me a sheaf of the holy lilies and a red pot filled with yellow roses for Rafik.

By the following morning the traveling flower-makers had gone onwards to other towns and villages of the Sierra Nevada. Colored drifts of snips of paper, bits of wire, piled mule dung and the charred-earth sphere of their night-time fire told of their resting-place. They had sold their wares well; many a Lanjaron child was to be seen in the town holding a Gypsy pot of flowers. The several wall shrines in and near Lanjaron were decorated with the white lilies; perhaps among them were several into which I had painted the yellow stripes.

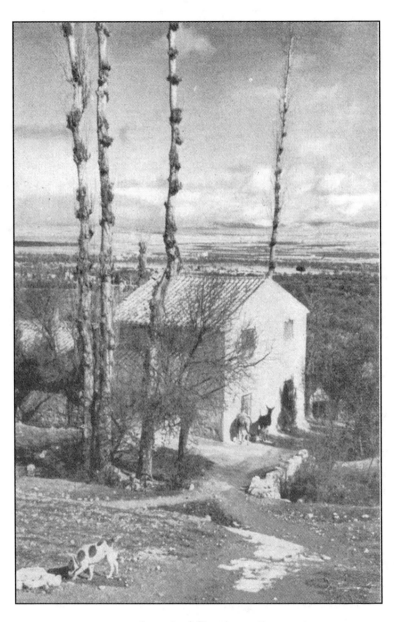

A typical Sierra *cortijo*.
Photo by Paul Stephenson

Chapter Seven

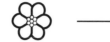

Journey in the High Sierra

Early in August and early in the morning, a man from the high Sierra Nevada came for me with his horse, and accompanied by Rafik, I began the long-desired journey to those mountain regions which for so long had tempted me from the water-mill. Now we became one of the procession of pack-carrying animals which, also, for so long I had watched from the mill terrace, seemingly moving always towards the blue sky which the mountain peaks clove like the steel-heads of axes.

From the very first paces that the horse took I experienced the discomfort of a sierra saddle. Fine enough to look upon with the embroidered girth and body bands and hanging woolen trappings of saffron and scarlet, but horrible to ride. The discomfort was caused by the bolster-like padding, which was used to prevent body sores caused by the heavy packs which the small sierra horses habitually carry to and from the mountain farms. On such a saddle one's legs are so spread apart that they stand sheer out from the horse on either side; and there are no stirrups.

All the morning, until early noon, the ride was straight up the mountain, and then it was followed by sheer down, which was the most difficult of all, with only one thin rein to help the difficult balancing. Furthermore, most of the time I had also to hold Rafik on the saddle in front of me, sideways, because his little legs could not go across the swaying saddle couch.

But the boy loved the riding and piped his excited exclamations like a blackbird almost throughout the journey, so that I thrust the discomfort to the back of my mind, and found much pleasure.

We rode before sun-up, and it was very cold. "Better the summer cold of the sierra than the summer heat," Juan, the guide, said. And when we did meet the full burn of the sun at midday, I saw that he spoke truly.

We rode much of the way behind a deaf man on a slow donkey, and there was no place on the narrow rocky track to pass in front of him. He shouted things back to me in friendliness, but, as he was totally deaf, he spoke a strange language which I did not understand, nor did Juan. I think that he was praising Rafik for sitting so valiantly on the jogging and slipping horse; Juan thought so too.

The track was very bad; only animals used to such travel could avoid slipping and cutting knees or breaking limbs. We rarely trod earth: for nearly all the journey the surface was bare rock, worn smooth and slippery as cobble-stones, worn thus by the feet of men and their animals which have gone to and from the mountain during its long history. There had been many sierra bandits, the guide said, and they were traveling the mountain not very long ago.

The lower slopes were shady with olive trees and chestnut. Small, hard berries were already showing on the olives, and round, green, almost hairy fruits containing the nuts crowded in remarkable abundance on the chestnuts. What appeared singular to me, and sad, was the number of ruined small ranches – the sierra *cortijos* – which we passed. Juan informed me that the people had abandoned them to live in the towns; the life on the upper sierra being very difficult, and in winter, terrible. And then nature had taken over the houses, and blown in roofs and battered down walls with her rampaging winds and rains of the high mountains.

However, the upper *cortijos* which we passed were mostly inhabited. Built of the gray stone of the sierra, they were squat weather-trammeled places, and their surrounding fruit trees and crops were stunted or spare, possessing none of the luxuriance of the lower fertile terraces where water was available.

Juan told me that in the spring the sierra blossomed with a thousand flowers. I was doubtful. I had walked the sierra in March and onwards and found nothing to compare with the mountains of Turkey, Mexico or North Africa, where indeed the wild flowers amazed the eyes and quickened the heart with the flash of their colors and their marvelous abundance.

The only flowers that I passed throughout the Sierra Nevada ride were lavender, rosemary and marjoram – those rich-scented sister plants – and foxgloves as tall as the horse which I was riding, so that we snipped off the rosy gloves as we rode by. Much ivy, then in fragrant flower, and a small white clematis, also of rich honey-scent, and the richest perfumed of all, the sulphur-hued broom, called *flor-de-Gallonba*, from which a pungent eau-de-cologne is made in Andalusia. There were also many of the shrubs which the Gypsies use for their basket-making and chair-weaving: *Rasea Vieja*, with the prickly leaves, and a form of willow, *Saa*. On one of the highest parts of the mountain I met with a Gypsy lad, a friend of mine, who had often carried Rafik on his back on long walks, Candido Castano. He had come the long distance alone, on foot, to gather the basket plants for his family.

After several hours of riding, the deaf man went away along a side-track and we had the mountain road clear before us and traveled towards the rising sun which lit the cold early morning sky with a Gypsy fiesta fire, flaming and wonderful.

At the first water-spring which we came to, we halted for breakfast, and Rafik and I waded in the icy stream which flowed from it, to take away the ache from our limbs. Despite the sun-heat the water touched cold as if ice crystals were within. The sierra journey was landmarked for me by the many fountains, especially Fuente Mato-marcas, Fuente Ventura, Fuente del Pinto.

The guide breakfasted simply, bread and cheese and wine, with walnuts; Rafik and I ate almost the same, but we drank the mountain water instead of wine and ate honey with our bread, which the guide did not like. Typical of many Spaniards and unlike the Arabs, he did not like sweet food of any kind, nor milk products with the exception of cheese. I remember when I first met Patrocinio, I presented her with a small bar of butter which I was carrying; she thought it was soap! She had never eaten butter in her sixty years.

Bread and cheese were the basis of our food for the journey, and for the rest, in typical sierra manner, we foraged as we rode by on crisp fresh onions, very young corn-cobs, wild watercress, and garbanzo – a small green legume, often sold ready boiled in the shops, also roasted and salted. The boiled chickpeas are much eaten by the poor-class families, since, for a few pence, one obtains a large dishful. From the trees we took young almonds and that delicious fruit *breviva,* which resembles a large black fig, but which ripens months earlier. As with figs, there is a white variety, but more rare; both taste like pure honey.

Juan declared no one minded travelers foraging a few handfuls of food here and there during journeys; it was only the filling of baskets, or the carrying away from the mountain of other people's toil and produce, which was considered a crime in the Sierra Nevada. Travelers mostly kept to the rules, but Juan informed me that nowadays there was an increase in cattle rustlers; therefore to protect the unfenced farms, guardians patrolled much of the mountain, and also the people mostly took their animals back to the town to sleep when they were only working their land daily and living away from the mountain. That accounted for the great trek of the animals at dusk and dawn, which Rafik and I, and even the baby, loved to meet and watch along the road which led to the town.

We saw no birds at all throughout the ride, not even around the fountains or in the olive groves: none. Juan said that on the highest ranges of the mountain, eagles lived, and they were bigger than the tall sierra men.

On the mountain also there is said to live that legendary lizard-animal of dragon-like appearance with a long tail: *lagarto*. It is described as being the friend of men, but the bitter enemy of women. It attacks, bites, and chases women away from the mountain. But the animal has a tremendous, almost magnetic, power to attract women, and for that reason young men are said to carry *lagartos* around concealed beneath jackets or even shirts. I met many people who said in all seriousness that they had seen this animal. Luz Perez told me that she had seen seven young ones at play.

"What did you do?" I asked.

"I fled away!"

From all the inhabited *cortijos* that we passed by, people came out to greet us, mostly to ask where we were going and to have us take messages of friendship from them to the other upper mountain-dwellers.

We ended our ride at a ranch close by the nurseries of the pine trees with which many of the upper stretches of the mountain were being planted, and close also to the waterfalls – grand and beautiful – which thundered down into the river passing tumultuously along the valley, a place of whirlpools and fathomless pits, and which in time, much tamed and depleted, came to the molino Gongoras.

This *cortijo* was called Del Pinto, and it was managed by a family of young people. The mother had died young in her fortieth year and the father was away managing another farm which the family owned. Two young women, Maria and Camella, were occupied preparing potatoes and runner beans for the midday meal. But they were happy to have visitors, and made places for us in the shade of a massive chestnut tree, the trunk of which was hollowed and made a cool sitting place. Rafik took delighted possession along with two kittens.

We sat and talked about the life of the sierra and also about the plague of typhus which was smiting people everywhere, but which seemed unable to reach the sierra heights that year. We talked in friendliness for about an hour, when Camella asked me if I would like to see the farm-house.

The low-built house was very old, old as the water-mill of Gongoras, I believe. Of rough gray sierra rock and stone, plastered and distempered within: across the ceiling chestnut beams of the same massive build as the shade-giving tree in the court. There was a big open fireplace with wood burning; over this a black iron pot was hung ready for the potatoes and runner beans which the sisters had been preparing, both much cultivated and popular foods on the sierra, especially the beans. Above the fireplace, which was certainly the heart of that small room, was nailed a large crucifix. There were many religious pictures on the wall, cheap-looking ill-printed things which mostly are purchased in the shops along with the groceries, or from stalls at the sierra fairs.

From the ceiling hung half a dozen bunches of *altabacca*, used to trap flies. I had thought that, on the high reaches of the mountain, the flies would have been left behind. But that had not proved to be so. All of the time that we had been sitting in the shade of the chestnut tree they had been afflicting us with their hissing and their stabbing stings, for the common house and field fly of the Sierra Nevada possesses a sting. The women told me that at night time the flies gathered on the bunches of *altabacca* to pass the night there, then the sierra people plunge the bunches into a sack and take the sack outside to the stream to drown the flies within it. That way they are able to sleep in peace even if by day they have to endure the molestation of the flies.

The bedroom was mostly possessed by a big square wooden bed built against the wall, like a wooden tray. Bedclothing was scattered across it. All the family shared that one bed, the men and the women. The pleasing thing in that room was a tiny window, set like a jewel in the wall, facing the bed. The mountain skies showed there, lapis lazuli background to the now-near mountain peaks.

The women gave us sweet red apples from their trees, and then we went to the water-holes to see if I could bathe in one or another of them. We passed by the threshing ground of the *cortijo*, where the brothers were amassing grain from the year's wheat, driving a fine pair of mules in the endless circling of the threshing ground.

It was a pleasant walk to the water-holes; the earth was so green along the trail of the water. But when we reached the holes they were just deep mud, bereft of water. The *cortijo* streams had been diverted to irrigate another farmer's lands. This sudden cutting-off of one's water supply must cause much annoyance to the sierra landowners, for, except during the short seasons of the rains, one could never be sure of enough water for one's work. Again and again the wheels of the water-mill were halted because there was insufficient water to turn them.

We sat once more in the tree shade, and the brothers came from their work, leading in the handsome mules which were tethered then to rings in the wall; buckets of water were placed beside the thirsty animals. The brothers joined the conversation now. All of the family were most handsome, with beautiful gray eyes set beneath very bushy brows (the women, too, had these eyebrows), abundance of hair, black as the farm cooking-pot, and lithe, muscular, long-limbed bodies.

One of the brothers was hump-backed, a great hump upon him, over which his shirt set in ugly shape. As usual with misshapen tragic people, we pretended not to notice anything. Rafik, with the innocently cruel eyes of a child, stared over-much; but he said nothing concerning that young man. Later, Juan told me that the youth had been injured in his fourteenth year. Until then there had been no sign of the hump on his back, and he had been – and still was – the best-looking of all that handsome family.

What cruel things life can do to one. Later I, too, was to bear the cross of physical ugliness: a very small one, but unpleasant, nevertheless. My cross was the loss of all of my hair. This is a typical result of severe typhus. I had never been told to expect this, although throughout typhus I had had an obsession concerning my hair. I must have felt it being burnt off at the roots by the terrible fever. The red-cloaked demon, typhus, did not take me, but he had my hair! It could be pulled out in handfuls like the hair from a doll, and in one month from the first sign of its falling, I had lost it all and had an almost completely bare head. I thus knew what it was like to be made ugly suddenly. Patrocinio wound my hair around her bunches of garlic stalks, and used it in her remedy to fume serpents out of the water-mill!

Early noon we left the hospitable and friendly company of the Cortijo del Pinto and turned back towards the water-mill. Rides home always seem longer than rides away: there is not the adventure of new places. Horses and human bodies are tired. And too, I was impatient to be with my baby again. A day away from her had seemed very long; and young though she was, I knew that she would be looking for me, which proved to be true. So the way back seemed very long and the fountains too far apart for our thirsty mouths.

The descent was much more difficult than the ascent. It was indeed like moving down a slippery staircase of rocks. The horse slipped, the saddle slipped, and Rafik went into a deep sleep, which meant that he possessed no balance at all. A hot wind came up and blew dust in our faces; it lay thick on hair and eyelashes and pricked our lips.

After an hour of such riding I told the guide that I must go on foot for all the further part of the journey back to the mill.

I soon acquired the foot-jog of the sierra people, necessary in order to make any progress down the slippery track of rock. I kept alongside the horse without difficulty.

The guide was not pleased to be on the horse and I on foot; but it was necessary for one of us to be mounted in order to support the sturdy body of Rafik, yet sleeping deeply from the long day in the rich air of the mountain heights.

It was not the first time that I had been on foot alongside a man mounted on a horse; there had been another time, but then it had been very different. On the Sierra Nevada the reason was necessity; not wishing to risk a fall from the horse during that sheer descent when so ill-balanced on that uncomfortable saddle, a bad fall very probably causing me to forfeit the care of my children again.

The other occasion had been on a mountain of northern Galilee on the border of Syria: the man on the horse had been a Bedouin Arab. And as I followed along the Sierra Nevada track, I recalled, in clear images, that time in Galilee.

Halid Abdullah, nephew of the great cattle-owning sheik, Abou Yussef, leader of the Toobah Bedouin Arabs, had been buying wine for his family in the Israeli village shop in Rosh Pinah. We met there, and he offered to take me back on his horse to the farm where I was working. I mounted behind Halid, on his Arab horse the creamy hue of a white rose, and on this creature, like a wild swan we sped over the sun-burnt earth. Halid wore a broad belt of black leather, studded with brass and embroidered with orange and purple wools; this I encircled with my hands around the slim waist. He was one of the most beautiful men I have met. To reach the farm we had to pass within sight of the black tents settlement of his people. And I, thinking for him, not for myself, for it was absolute happiness on the horse, suggested that for the rest of the way I should walk, so as not to annoy his Bedouin wives through his riding with a European woman. So for quite a distance I had followed behind the Arab's horse: over hot stony earth crowded with great barbed thistles and thorns, the former which scorched my feet through my thin sandals, the latter which tore at my legs and dress. But I had walked in joy, telling myself: "This Bedouin I could follow to the end of the world!"

Nearing the finish of the Sierra Nevada ride we met with a party of men who were friends of Juan. They were seated like Gypsies around a big fire, a frying-pan filled with sliced potatoes in olive oil, cooking there. The hot, pleasing scent came to us as we rode up to the fire. Rafik woke from his sleep; the scent of the potatoes and the high voices of the men enticed him back into the sierra world. The men, again Gypsy-like, were near a stream of water, and the child took off his sandals and splashed in contentment in the cool coursing water.

These friends of the guide had time to sit around a fire and fry potatoes. One of them was a water-man, in charge of the sierra streams, keeping them free from down-washed stone and wrack and weeds, and diverting water for irrigation of the lands around and below the streams. Another was a guardian of the sierra, to protect the unfenced lands of the farms from pillagers of the animals and crops, also to protect the wild animal life of the mountain from over-greedy hunting. The other two men were shepherds, then without work, now that the spring and summer pasturing on the mountain was already ended, the months of fierce sun having scorched everywhere any distance from the streams.

We sat down with the men and accepted some of their potatoes. When these were all eaten, the fire was beaten out, and a bottle of wine shared, and all turned their time to the exchanging and the singing of Sierra Nevada songs, for my pleasure. Poetically worded songs about shepherd love, family feuds, adventuring of the bygone bandits, and mountain life. There were no songs of soldiering or war sung in that peaceful grove, murmurous with the breeze-stirred olive-trees' foliage and sun-dried grasses and wild lavender.

I filled my pockets and Rafik's pockets and one of my saddlebags with heads of the lavender, and my hands and wrists became fragrant with the sweet and pungent flower perfume which the sun had not been able to dry into nothingness.

We stayed over an hour and then we thanked the men for the pleasure that we had known with them around the stream-side fire, and we moved on again. My limbs were rested from that tiresome saddle, so I mounted the horse a further time, and held once more in my arms the sturdy little body of Rafik, now sweet and fresh from his time in the stream, for he had taken off his clothes also and bathed there.

We gathered some more *breviva* fruits and almonds and the very first of the prickly cactus fruits, for they – the famed wild *chumbas* of the Sierra Nevada – were only just opening.

Soon we came within sight of the river swimming-pool where I had so often swum, and I knew then that the water-mill of Gongoras was near.

The beauty of the last stretch of the long ride was memorable, for we had ridden into the evening, and the mountains had turned the purple-blue of Indian lilac, and the sun was setting into a sky color flecked and brilliant as a peacock's tail. The river was a lavender ribbon against the dark flanks of the mountain and its color recalled to me the harvest of lavender heads that I carried in my pockets and in the saddle-bag. I told myself that I would make a sachet of the flowers for the baby's cradle as a gift to her from the high Sierra Nevada.

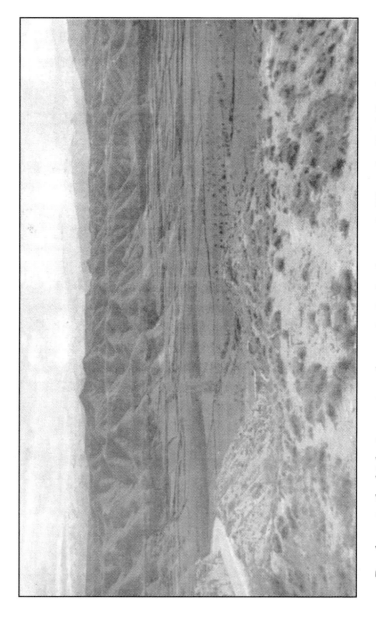

Roadway to the high sierra; eternal snow in the background. Photo by Paul Stephenson

Chapter Eight

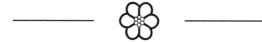

We Leave The Mountain

The mountain was never before so rich to my eyes as during the months of autumn into early winter. There was such a profound ripening: even the great harvest moons were a splendid gold.

The maize was almost all cut and was being ripened in house-yards, on the now tranquil threshing grounds, and on the roofs of many small country dwellings. I think that of all the daubed artist's palette of color which I saw on the Sierra Nevada, the maize cobs ripening in the hot autumn sun pleased my eyes the most. Such an intense orange color, more brilliant even than the wild marigolds which the rains were bringing into flower again after their long dying since the time of the spring and summer heats and parched earth. I think the only comparable thing were the pistils of the autumn crocuses, the saffron from which flowers came the brilliant dye of Spanish rice.

The rains which came over the mountain were not gentle. They came companioned by fierce winds. They blew away the wide-brimmed straw hats of the sierra men, which had given shade against the blaze of the sun on the mountain, and soon the straw hats were being replaced by the drabber felt ones and tight-fitting berets, which I had seen worn when I arrived on the mountain in the early spring.

Especially the winds flung down the fruits which clustered in such abundance on the chestnut and walnut trees of the sierra.

There are things to tell about the chestnuts and walnuts of the mountain.

One of my favorite Gypsy families were the Castanos – chestnut trees, who married with the Cerezas – cherry trees. Their children were beautiful. They dealt in poultry and pigeons. The sale of the pigeons for food was a particularly sad thing, for they are such fair and gentle birds and fly into so many Spanish love songs, especially the old songs of Spain.

Roasted chestnuts are an important autumn-time food of the people of the mountain. Many people prepare them in their own homes, roasting them in sieves over their brazier charcoal fires. But many also purchase them already roasted from the chestnut-sellers, who are found in all the mountain villages, sitting at street corners by their glowing braziers, perfuming all the air around with the rich scent of the roasting nuts. They possessed wooden mallets and also knives and cans of salt. The nuts were hit with the mallet to soften their shells, and then split with a knife and salt rubbed in to speed the roasting, and give whiteness and extra flavor.

Those chestnut-sellers, amusingly, seemed from the same family: all of them stout, aged women, clad in black, white aproned, smeared with charcoal. But, like many families, there were the good and the bad among them. The good sold beautiful nuts, the bad mixed with the fresh nuts the stale old ones from the previous days' roastings. I soon came to know those of the sellers from whom to buy the good quantity of chestnuts which Rafik and I ate daily; and a little of which the baby had also, pounded into flour and mixed into her goat milk when she took her meals from a cup. Indeed, late into November, roast chestnuts were the basis of our evening meal, together with fresh white grapes and wheaten bread; we ate little else. For mid-day we often had *batatas*: a long beetroot-like tuber, yellow of flesh, which tasted of chestnuts. I expect that it was this form of the potato which was used as a typhus treatment in the ancient Mexican army. During the Spanish Civil War, the soldiers of both sides often lived for weeks on chestnuts, I was told, especially so around the mountains of the Sierra Nevada.

I had seen the chestnut trees of that mountain in first leaf, bright from their unaccustomed bathing by the springtime snow. I had seen the chestnut flowers, foamy and creamy as the river spume, and enjoyed their lovely far-reaching scent. I had watched the pale wands of those flowers turn to tarnished gold, whereon they fell in golden rain from the trees, to be gathered, when sun-dried, by Gypsy children from the families of basket-weavers – the children to give practice to their young hands by turning the tassels of flowers into little nests for the frightened weeping bird fledglings which they plundered from the parent nests. I had seen the fruits form, pale green spheres, prickly as a hedgehog's back, making dapples of emerald on the green-black body of the foliage. Then, when time and the autumn sunlight had ripened the fruits, turning them from green to brown, came the winds and blew them from the boughs, so tired with their heavy bearing, ready for the braziers of the chestnut-roasters. It was part of Spanish autumn life to walk out in the cold misty evenings and buy the hot sweet fruits and burn one's hands and lips in the good eating. Later Rafik and I learned to roast them on our own brazier. But by mid-December that rich and healthful harvest was ended and it was difficult to come by any nuts at all.

The walnuts gave me a new herbal treatment. I had rammed a rose-thorn down a fingernail when gathering rose hips for syrup for the baby. This had turned septic, and I could not find any of the herbs that I wanted for its cure. Peasants told me to pulp up walnut hearts when the nuts were still young on the tree, and to apply the pulp around my finger, keeping it in position with a cotton cloth soaked in vinegar. In half a day pus had pressed up out of the nail, and my painful finger was cured. Two other cures they told me for my finger were: rubbing live wood-lice into the sore area, or human milk, the latter also a cure for earache.

The walnut trees were also associated with an adventure which came to Rafik. Two big trees dropped their fruits alongside a part of the path near the swimming-pool. Every morning on the walk to the pool I collected nuts for Rafik. One morning I had collected a small heap of nuts and was occupied cracking them with a flint, when I heard a man's voice shouting in great fear. I looked up to see a cow almost upon my little son, who was standing on a narrow arch over the pathside stream, throwing stones into the water. The cow was one of those huge animals from the high sierra, about as large as a Friesian bull. She had wandered down alone from the mountain. There was no room for the cow and the child on that bridge: he would either be trampled upon or pushed into the stream where he surely would be injured against one of the boulders. I was too far away to reach Rafik before the cow! The great beast came upon the child, knocked him with her head into a sitting position and then stepped over him, flicking his face with her tail as she walked away.

The little boy shouted joyfully: "Cow! Cow!"

Can one's heart tremble? Mine trembled!

The miller from the Paraisio mill, who had shouted the warning, came running to me. "What good fortune!" he cried. "I thought your child would be killed."

I told him then, "The cow didn't hurt him because she knew that we love her people and do not eat them or any other animals."

I spoke somewhat defiantly. For a large sow, shut in perpetual darkness in a small building of the mill which I passed daily, used to pain me. The world all those days was golden with sunlight, but the sow never knew the sun, except her snout which she thrust longingly beneath the tread of the door where the snout had scraped a hollow place. Sometimes her neighbor, the walnut tree, tossed an odd nut to her. What joy such notice from the tree must have been to her in that imprisoned Lady-of-Shalott life.

The autumn harvest of the molino Gongoras, garnered by the miller's wife, increased weekly in quantity and beauty. Green and red peppers were split open, salted, and set to dry alongside the tomatoes; they resembled little red and green canoes. Peaches were quartered and added to the drying things, also almonds, shelled and salted. The scent was magnificent. All the lesser scents mingled to make a pungent perfume of healthful sun-drenched food. How different from the stench of animal paunches and intestines being washed in the surrounding streams and the river.

The pleasure of Patrocinio's terrace harvest was spoiled for me by swarming wasps. The viciousness of these wasps was an experience new to me! They possessed much of the aggressive devilry of the Sierra Nevada flies. Perhaps more devilry! – for they stung so severely. As one walked by the terrace they swooped upon one like dive-bombers and stung. The stings possessed the viciousness of the stingers and swelled up big as oranges and irritated for a week or more. Patrocinio said that wasp stings were good for one's health and those who were stung were lucky! She could have had all the wasp luck which came to Rafik and me. Fortunately the baby was never stung, never felt those intensely painful stings.

My own harvest of tomatoes and figs and walnuts was stored away in a sack ready for our traveling, for we were leaving the water-mill before the winter properly came over the mountain.

As usually happens to me when I am having to leave a place which I have loved, things occurred to lessen my sorrow of departure. The ants in my room had become terrible; they were ready to enter everything immediately if vigilance was relaxed. I kept them away with powdered pyrethrum flowers – which pungent scent they hated, and indeed were slain by its pungency. Baskets holding flour, raisins and fruit had to be hung from the roof on chains. But during the last few weeks at the mill, the ants even found their way down the chains and I found the flour seething with them: therefore paraffin rags had to be applied and renewed daily, tainting my hands with that horrible smell.

The great black ants nested above a far wall of my room. They had to be kept back also by pyrethrum flung against the wall, or lemon peel rubbed there on the rough plaster. This all took more time than I cared to spare, for I had the sole care of the two small children, a book to be written, and a great deal of herbal correspondence always reaching me. Days came when I had not the time to apply such things, and then the insects invariably came forward in triumph and cost me more hours of my day than ever.

The salamanders also had become a nuisance. When I had first come to the mill they had been but a pair in my room there, and had amused me with the antics of their supple dragon-shaped bodies of over half a foot long, the unmoving eyes with which they fixed me and their strange-sounding voices which were company during the nights. But a family had been reared and that troupe of young ones were like demons in a pantomime, who leap up onto the stage from trap-doors in the floor, or descend on invisible wires from the roof; the salamanders frequently leapt out at me from unexpected hiding-places.

During my last weeks in the water-mill there must have been a late hatching of a family of Red Admiral butterflies, for six times young salamanders danced triumphantly on the walls of my room, carrying in their mouths the fluttering butterflies. What a sadness! The salamanders moved too quickly when I tried to catch them to rescue their victims. There is an Andalusian belief that if one drinks the water in which a salamander has fallen, all one's hair will fall out. I heard that a while before I developed typhus. I seemed destined to lose my hair one way or another! For, apart from the typhus, there were many salamanders, like jacks-in-the-box, leaping into my days and nights – especially the nights.

One of my most powerful memories of that autumn on the mountain was my falling hair. Not in strands was it falling, but in pitiful handfuls. I had thought at times that I would save some of it. But by the late autumn, I knew that its loss was inevitable: As sure as the chestnut leaves being blown from the trees by the sierra winds and leaving bare boughs, my hair would go.

Patrocinio was angry that I was leaving the mill. People who knew her well warned me that she would exert all her powers to keep me there. I think she would not have been angered if I had been going away from Spain altogether, to England or Turkey. But she knew that I was moving to another part of Spain, taking the children away to the sea. I told her truthfully that I needed the sea: the love of it was in my heart. My father had come from the Turkish port of Smyrna, my mother from Egypt's Alexandria. I possess a beautiful spiked white shell which I had found on the sands of Tetuan in Spanish Morocco (I have never seen another shell like it there or on any other coast); when I am far from the sea and I long for it, I can hold the shell to my ear and hear the recording of the sea's murmur. The children love that murmuring too. Rafik certainly; he had been born on a sea island, and Luz seemed to like it, too.

Luz by late autumn had grown into a beloved personality, and everyone told me that she was beautiful. I could not judge myself, seeing near perfection in most things that I greatly love! But, in true fact, the baby much reminded me of a cook who had worked for us in the now seemingly far-away days of my childhood: a prim old-fashioned woman. Indeed Rafik and I called the baby that name: Lucy Hunt.

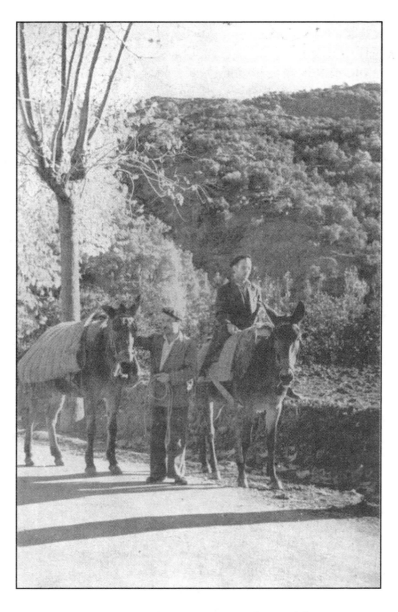

Sierra Nevada mules, showing the woolen saddle trappings
and broad saddles without stirrups.
Photo by Juan Mingorance

"Loochi Hant, Loochi Hant!" piped Rafik, in his peculiar Spanish-type English. We also called her *Rosa de España* – the Rose of Spain.

One of my preparations for leaving, apart from the sun-dried fruits, was the buying of a large quantity of honey – honey of the mountain, where the bees were semi-wild and the honey was gathered and stored, all naturally. In Lanjaron, in the main street, there was a honey woman. This honey woman kept her sweet stock in huge stone jars, quite the size of those in which hid the forty thieves of the Aladdin legend. In place of the thieves was stored the honey of many kinds, from the mountain. My favorite was a thick sand-colored variety which was said to be chestnut blossom. I needed much honey for the baby.

It was about that time that I bought for Rafik an Andalusian book of legends. In it was the Spanish legend of the Milky Way, the prince who was fed by a goat. In that version of the legend there was an important addition. The prince was reared on goat's milk and honey! That brought Luz closer than ever to the legend. For she was always given honey after her drinks of goat's milk. The doctor had not wanted honey for the baby (nor had he wanted goat's milk indeed, preferring her to have some modern dried milk product). He said that honey was too strong and too fermentative a food. [Ed. note: Honey can contain spores of the organism that causes botulism, a deadly poison; however, only babies under a year old are at risk.] But I knew that honey was precious substance for the baby; it even told so in the Bible, and there in that Andalusian legend I found that the Oriental prince had also been reared that way!

I think that I loved the mountain best in the autumn, perhaps because I was leaving it very soon, and then also nearly having lost through typhus the right to look again upon any mountain of the earth, I appreciated it the more. Its splendor that autumn seemed never to have been surpassed,

Spanish Mountain Life

not even at the time of the nightingales. The maize was a delight to me. The field of my neighbor had been sown late. Most of the Sierra Nevada maize had been cut already and was drying in ochre beauty all around the area of the watermill. Day and night I had at my side the song of the ripening maize in the field against my wall. Not a whispering and whimpering as with the wheat, but a kind of primitive war or marching song. The long flat leaves slapped each other when the winds blew them, and they slapped also the heavy cobs. How bright were those leaves in the light of sun and moon! and how tall the maize had grown! There were yet flowers on many of the plants along with the cobs; they grew on separate stalks opening out into fans of silver feathers on which goldfinches rested and were rocked by the maize plant. I cut one plant and it reached to the ceiling of my room, and was a thing of joy for Rafik and me until the ants invaded it, and then we fed the cobs to the goat and ate some ourselves, raw, spread lightly with oil of sweet almonds.

The lizards who inhabited the terrace suddenly grew emerald tails, whereas hitherto, only days ago, they were all a drab dust-brown. I believe that the green was protective coloring, preparing for the green time which was coming quickly with the winter rains. The lizards had become used to the children and me on their terrace, and sometimes sped across our feet or arms.

Everyone at this time was talking about the Sierra Nevada fairs. Before the coming of winter, fairs were held at many towns and villages of that mountain range: the main purpose being selling off of surplus animals and celebration of the harvest, with wine and song. The fairs were always great occasions for the Gypsies, who rode in small covered wagons from one fair to another, their men being prominent in the animal barter and the women, for the time being, becoming professional entertainers of dancing and fortune-telling. The Gypsies wore traditional picturesque costumes, and the men also put on a matador-like *Emery* to give their part in entertainment with guitar and mandolin, their fine tenor voices soaring in flamenco song.

I had planned to visit Orgiva fair with Maria and Rosario, as that town was the nearest fair close to Lanjaron. Further away was the fair of Montril. It was a three-day fiesta at Orgiva. But one's plans do not always end in fulfillment. Increasing trouble at the water-mill made me decide not to stay for the fair. It was not a very sad decision for me to make. It would have hurt me seeing all the animals assembled for sale, mostly for slaughter; I would be greeted by sheep I'd herded and by many of the individual sheep and goats with which my child and I had become acquainted.

Rosario, the Gypsy who had fostered Luz for a while, came to wish me farewell. She came the day before I left and helped me with the washing. She also brought buckets of water for me from the quite distant fountain. I had been doing likewise until my arms would obey my wishes no longer, they ached so much. Going very late for water on one of my last nights, I met Juan the Gypsy, one of the basket weavers and popular for his fine voice, but a rather fat and disheveled man and no figure of romance. Yet that night he did create romance around him, for there he was at that late hour, alone, washing himself at the fountain by the light of the moon, his long hair dripping with silvered water and his flesh gleaming.

It had become increasingly necessary for me to collect my own water supplies, for the miller's wife was cheating again, and bringing me polluted water from the near streams instead of from the safe fountain flow. I had found in my bucket the tiny black worms which live fastened to the herbage of dirty water. I had challenged her and we had had one of our angry "exchanges." Those quarrels with Patrocinio became very frequent during my last weeks. Once she saw that I was packing trunks and knew that, positively, I was leaving the mill, she was more short-tempered even than formerly.

I had a presentiment that one or other of the children would meet with a fatality before we were all away from the mill. Rafik might fall down one of those terrible tunnels of the water-mill into which the waters roared and foamed, and about which all of my friends had warned me when visiting me in the garden of the upper stream. Luz might get a snake in her basket. I myself at that time had slipped on the rock steps going up to the terrace, a thing which had never happened before, not even during typhus when my limbs were so weak. I had nearly cut my skull across during that fall. I would not let the children out of my eyes or those of my Gypsy friends who came to help me, and it was all very difficult. I felt besieged.

The Gypsies came in a crowd to wish me good luck.

Rosario's remarkable mother, Angustia, came among them. A very tall woman with a finely modeled Native American Indian form of face and figure, and with dark, liquid – almost sad – eyes. False eyes! There was little sad about that woman. She was the Great Beggar (*Bauro monger*). During that summer and autumn tourist season she constantly wore a bandage around one of her chestnut-brown, scraggy legs; and she would monger for pesetas for her wound – beneath the bandage – which she declared she was too deprived of money to be able to cure! I asked Rosario about the wound. She said that it was painted there! a daub of blue and red paint, nothing more.

Angustia strode into the garden of the water-mill; very soon her pockets bulged with quince fruits and tomatoes. I had not seen the Gypsy in action, but I was glad for Patrocinio to experience a little of what she inflicted upon others.

That was my last afternoon in the mill garden. I was very tired at that time from a night of packing. For there were not only the clothes, but big quantities of my books, and reference books, quantities of herbs, and Rafik's cheap toys, none of which he would let me leave behind. I had not space for everything and had to flow over into baskets which the Gypsies supplied. That noon I longed to sit quietly in the sun. I could have sat tranquilly enough with my friends Rosario and Maria, but the other Gypsies were there, mother and relatives of Rosario. Almost all of my Gypsy visitors that noon were black-clad. For in a similar way to their neighbors, the Portuguese Gypsies seemed to mourn distant relatives for years.

They chattered as tirelessly as starlings on winter evenings, and all the time Rosario's mother was mongering: "Would I not be taking this and that with me?"

"All! All!" I finally shouted at her, ending politeness.

I had already given away everything which I did not need. Rosario was happy for I had presented her with Rafik's big out-of-doors earthenware bath and she was to have my bucket when I left.

This had angered the miller's wife; for she had coveted those two things although she knew that both were long promised to the Gypsy. That was especially why she coveted; the bucket might have been made of gold she wanted it so much. But I would not be talked out of any promise spoken. This was a thing that I had learned impressively from my father: it was important and I was teaching it to my children.

Rosario's mother did a thing which was to have some significance later. She lifted up the three small bells which I had tied, on a ribbon, to Luz's basket. The baby loved to play with them; when she was hungry, often enough she would ring her bells! Rafik had worn them on his jacket when we had lived in England's New Forest. The bells used to tell me where he was in the forest, for much before his second year he wandered far. They were worth only a few pence but of much family value to me. Angustia lifted up the bells in her tawny clutching fingers and spoke quickly to Rosario.

"They are my baby's lucky bells," I said sharply, and without pulling unduly had the bells out of the mongering hands.

At that time Patrocinio appeared with her son and ally Rafael.

"Move quickly," she said. "The land is being irrigated!" She was visiting a petty triumph over the Gypsies and me especially me, for she knew how much I enjoyed sitting in the sun in the quiet of the garden. Indeed my whole day was a rush of work to achieve that pleasure.

There was no urgency to irrigate the garden that day. Rains had fallen recently, and on the morrow I was leaving. I had paid her very well for much of one year; over-paid her, my Spanish friends said. Having made the announcement the miller's wife and her son then walked away. I sat in silence for a while, and watched the muddy water creeping towards my island in the sun. Then I asked Rosario and Maria to come quickly with me, and Rafik too, for I wanted him to see what was going to be done.

I spoke with the Gypsy girls, and then they laughed and the three of us raced to the place where the bank of the upper mill-stream was opened to let out the stream waters for the irrigation. Straining our arms and our bodies we dragged heavy stones and boulders into the opening and quite closed it up. The waters were thus all pushed back to the end of the garden, and my sitting-place, where there was also shade for the baby's cradle, was left quite dry, and we went back to be in the sun again. The other Gypsies left us then, and soon Rosario also, and only the gentle Maria stayed with her small son, Pepe, who was Rafik's friend.

I occupied myself in memorizing the garden and the facing mountain. I even dared to look well at the cemetery across the maize field, now that I was going away safely.

I missed the swallows flying around me: they had left the mountain sooner than I. Always the swallows seemed to my mind to personify the attar of freedom. They come to places and go away, when they choose. They travel freely without passports and nonsense. Yes, they go when they care, and never stay to tell anyone or to ask permission, and yet all those places where they visit, the human population would have had them stay, for they not only personify freedom but also the warmth of spring and summer, and love in the sun, and ripening grain and fruits. But they can not be kept in cages in human houses: they die. So they are left unmolested.

Patrocinio returned to the garden to collect tomatoes. She saw then what had happened to her irrigation. By the time she had gathered her fruits and was ready for argument, the children and I had left the garden.

Late in the evening the miller and his wife came with an offering of dried figs and walnuts. I accepted both and gave Patrocinio two baskets and some of the baby's toys for her grandchild.

The following morning, soon before my departure, Rosario arrived, and seeing the figs and nuts warned me not to take them away with me, wanting me to return them to Patrocinio. For, she said, they had been given with bad feelings and would "grow beasts in them."

I did not accept her warning, and she proved to be right. The bad feeling had been mostly with the figs, for it was a quantity of them that Patrocinio had wanted to trade with me for my bucket, though I did not tell that to the Gypsy. There had been no trouble ever with the miller. From the day of my arrival at his mill to the very end, he had always been both friend and help to both my children and me; a quiet good man.

The walnuts were a success and later Rafik passed hours cracking and eating Sierra Nevada walnuts, far from the mountain, on the sands beyond Malaga. The figs, however, "grew beasts!" Only a few weeks after I possessed them I found great fat pink grubs crawling out from the head of the sack wherein the figs were stored above the sun-dried tomatoes. The tomatoes which I had purchased and dried myself, a half hundredweight, were untouched. I fed all Patrocinio's figs to the chickens.

Rosario was further of much help to me that busy last morning, carrying heavy luggage to the wagon, keeping the two children amused. But she was in my room for one intention, to steal my baby's bells, for certain on the orders of her mother.

She stole Luz's bells, all three of them! Unfortunately it was not until we were half a day's ride from the mountain that we discovered the loss, otherwise I would have returned to have them back from her.

My friend Luz Perez was traveling with me as far as Malaga, and during the ride she told me an Andalusian superstition concerning Spanish Gypsies – especially those of the Sierra Nevada. Such Gypsies possess an inherited lust for bells, she said, which are thought by them to hold much good luck, and according to their superstition, stolen bells were luckiest of all. No bell was safe from them: from church bells to those worn by animals. My own link with the Gypsies was proved to me yet further by that event. For I had decorated my children and my goat-like Afghan hounds, with bells long before I knew that it was a rite shared by the Spanish Gypsies. I recalled a Spanish Gypsy song, wherein as part of a Gypsy woman's beauty, as sung by her lovers, was the possession of forty *cascabelos* (little bells).

The goat was milked dry for my baby, just before we departed, to have the milk as fresh as possible for the day's traveling.

When the actual moment of departure came, Patrocinio wept. I wept later! only for the goat. I had wanted to take her away with me, and then later to England and Turkey – Luz's gentle black mother. Several letters had been written to the agricultural officials in England. But entry for the animal into England had been refused. My sadness was only tempered by the fact that it would have been difficult for me: traveling with two young children and a goat.

I was very worried about her, wondering as to her feelings at the sudden ending of her feeds for my baby. To lessen the goat's sadness, Luz was given her drinks of milk with cup and spoon, and was taken to see the goat at all of her former feeding times, with gifts of the animal's favorite foods: from beans and wheaten bread to grapes and figs.

On almost all of my travels I had known pain at having to leave behind an animal because of the British Isles animal quarantine laws, which have long seemed to me to be presumptuous where milch animals are concerned when considering the amount of animal disease in England at the present day resulting from unnatural rearing. Now I wept over Salud the goat, and held her to me, deeply hurt at the enforced separation.

"Be kind to her," I said tearfully and tritely. "Pet her and talk to her, she wants both those things. And don't let Fraquito beat her or tie up her ear tight against her horn." The latter was done to discipline the animal; it was defended, and was customary on the sierra. But I never saw such done beyond the water-mill.

Both the miller and his wife were good to the goat, but she was, in actual fact, owned by the elder son, Fraquito. He was a likeable man and kind with all children, but when he was in an ill humor – which was over-frequently – he burnt out his red temper on the goat. I had intervened and had protected her many times.

The neighbors crowded around the children and me, wishing us a good journey. Rosario and Maria rode in the coach with us to the outskirts of the town. We traveled early and thus met with the morning procession of the animals going forth to the mountain grazing. Away from the Sierra

Spanish Mountain Life

Nevada I would miss that music of swinging collar bells and hastening feet.

As we went past the baker's, the pungent scent of rosemary wood came across the town from the chimneys and I was reminded of my first day on the mountain, when that scent had pleased me. How truly it was typical of the mountain: a fragrant ancient custom. Not very practical as a modern fuel, but worth retaining for always, because it gave a sweet taste to Spanish bread, especially that which is made of wheat and maize grown on the Sierra Nevada and ground into flour by one or other of its ancient water-mills.

We traveled a whole morning and half a noon away from the sierra to the sea, where we found a new home on the sands, part of a very old inn set between two great rocks. There we found ourselves with very good-hearted Spanish people and had the further happiness of flamenco guitar music and song for much of the day and late into the evening, for the owner of the inn, Miguel Cerdan, justifiably possessed some fame for his music and people gathered to hear him, though often he played and sang just for his own pleasure. Dolphins chased fish in the blue sea and sported there also, leaping and plunging in beautiful rhythm; slowly they were moving away south, sensing winter's coming. Of the same mind as the dolphins were skeins of wild gray geese, who in typical and thrilling manner honked across the brilliant sky when the moon was waxen full, wanting near Africa. There were fleas in my room, they kept me awake; and therefore I was helped to finish the writing of my book about Spanish Mountain Life.

The evenings and nights, as November came, turned cold as soon as the wonderful winter sun dropped behind the hills, and we had braziers in our room again. We seemed to be seeing through the cycle of the year in Spain. I found an old tin, and had a fisherman make holes in it to form a sieve, and therein we roasted excellent Spanish chestnuts nightly. I asked the shopkeeper from where had come the chestnuts?

And I was told, "The Sierra Nevada!"

And then oh! one clear morning in late November, I saw a distant mountain peak across the bay towards Almeria, pointing up high above the Malaga range. Upon it lay snow shaped like the white, face-concealing hoods of the penitentes who paraded in the Semana Santa processions of Lanjaron last April. Yes, that was how it looked to me; and I asked the fishermen about that peak upon which the early snow had settled. They told me: "The Sierra Nevada."

The naming quickened my heart, for such a company of memories were then aroused at seeing the mountain again, it was as if a company of the wild geese had reversed their flight and come winging back upon me.

By that time much of the pain and horror which I had known upon the mountain had gone from my mind. I remembered mostly the nightingales and the Gypsies, I think. Both the children were strong and well. Rafik played in the fishing-boats the day long, and became an active member of a pack of wild and unruly fisher-children whom he loved.

Luz had become fat and brown and sweet as a Spanish chestnut, whereas before, after her illness, she had resembled a may-fly for frailness, those gossamer insects which live and dance for only one day and then die. She had her own particular cow, an immense black and white animal named Florentina, as successor to Salud the goat of our mountain life. Every morning at sunrise I ran a mile along the sands to a tiny fisherman's house where the big cow lived, and brought back a quart of milk, warm and spumey.

I, too, was strong again, and sun-dark, and my hair was growing. I possessed a black crop of hair now, like a man, and could walk again in the streets without occasioning too much interest and comment, such as I had had to endure before. But all its former silkiness seemed to have been lost, and the new hair was pressing up from my scalp wiry and ugly. That I had to accept, the wiry, ugly hair. I was thankful to be alive and enjoying life with my children.

People could say that I was to blame for what had happened on the mountain, that I should never have gone to such a primitive place. But I am not the first traveler to be stricken with a fever in Spain; one is always wiser after the pains of life. So whenever I looked across the bay to the Sierra Nevada with new snow upon its rocky and Gypsy-dark brow, I knew no bitterness at all, and felt mostly thankfulness for what I had seen and learned there: my love for Spain, my belief in herbs, all strengthened by my experiences on the mountain.

Most of that I was writing into my book – but not quite all. A head of wild lavender which I had brought back from the high sierra marked the pages of my copy-book as I wrote laboriously in pencil, keeping one ear listening towards where Luz lay in her Gypsy cradle, my baby of the Sierra Nevada. My other ear: to where Miguel was seated in the doorway of his inn, making endless music on his rich-toned old guitar, and also very often singing in flamenco-style, songs of many things: of departures and far journeys, Gypsies and cascabelos, love and lullabies, funerals and fiesta.

Copyright Notice

Acknowledgments

For the current edition, © 2011

A Gypsy wink and a big basket of thanks to the wise women who made this book a reality:

- **Jane Bond** and **Kimberly Eve** for turning Juliette's words into electrons.
- **Kimberly Eve** for her wonderful cover illustrations, interior illustrations and design skills.
- **Jennifer Jo Stevens** for seeing to the never-ending details: the quotes, the numbers, the codes, the facts.
- **Betsy Grace Sandlin**, best friend of words and guardian of the commas.
- **Rose Weissman**, for diligent, delightful assistance.
- **Rev. Ursula Carrie Wilkerson** for scanning photos.
- **Andrea Dworkin** for design assistance.
- **Susun Weed**, for typesetting, editing, designing, and keeping it all humming along.
- Our **guardians**, **grandmothers**, **spirit sisters**, and the **Ancient Ones**.

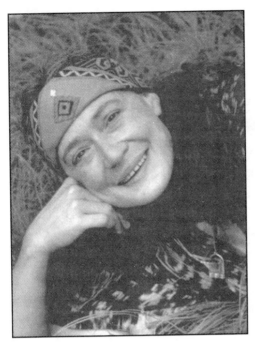

Susun S. Weed (left), editor-in-chief of Ash Tree Publishing, shamanic herbalist, goatkeeper, and lover of women, is thrilled to have this chance to bring Juliette's words and wisdom to the current generation of herbalists.

Kimberly Eve (right) is head of the art department and chief artist at Ash Tree Publishing. She has worked to bring several of Juliette's books back into print.

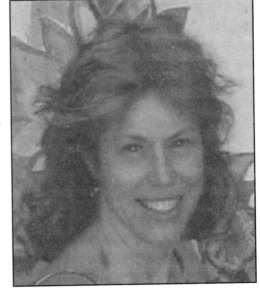

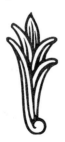

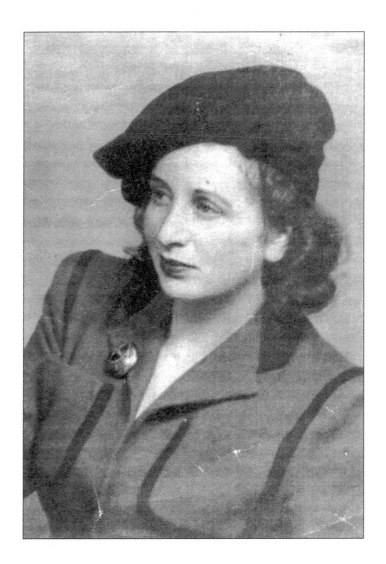

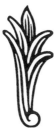  **Juliette de Bairacli Levy** (1911–2009) is honored as the grandmother of modern American herbalism. She has devoted her life to the health and well being of domesticated animals, especially dogs. Her herbals and memoirs have been in print, and in use, for over fifty years.

Other books you will want to read from

Ash Tree Publishing
Women's Health, Women's Spirituality

Wise Woman Herbal Series
best-sellers by
Susun S Weed

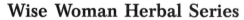

Herbals of Our Foremothers Series
classics by
Juliette de Bairacli Levy

and, by **Maida Silverman**

To order:

• Visit www.wisewomanbookshop.com
• Write to PO Box 64, Woodstock, NY 12498

Prices subject to change.